16.96

SURVIVING
HEALTHCARE

SURVIVING
HEALTHCARE

How to Take Charge And Get The Best
From Your Doctor, Your Hospital And
Your Health Insurance

Pamela Armstrong, MPH, MBA

CHESTNUT RIDGE BOOKS

Chestnut Ridge Books • Concord, CA

Published by: Chestnut Ridge Books
2269 Chestnut Street, #119
San Francisco, CA 94123-2600, USA

info@SurvivingHealthcare.com

SURVIVING HEALTHCARE
Pamela Armstrong

Armstrong, Pam.

Surviving healthcare / Pam Armstrong. -- 1st ed. -- Concord, CA : Chestnut Ridge Books, 2004.

p. ; cm.

ISBN: 0-9754560-5-9

1. Medical care--United States--Evaluation. 2. Public health--United States--Citizen participation. 3. Consumer education.
I. Title.

RA399.A3 A76 2004
362.1/0973--dc22   0409

Book Design by Pamela Terry, Opus 1 Design
Editor: Brookes Nohlgren
Cartoon Illustrator: Peter Winter

Printed in Canada

10 9 8 7 6 5 4 3 2 1
First Edition

Americans should be able to count on receiving care that meets their needs and is based on the best scientific knowledge. Yet there is strong evidence that this frequently is not the case.... Quality problems are everywhere, affecting many patients. Between the healthcare we have and the care we could have lies not just a gap, but a chasm.

From the Executive Summary, Institute of Medicine,
Crossing the Quality Chasm

Acknowledgments

Many people helped me in the process of writing *Surviving Healthcare*. I am profoundly grateful to every one of them.

First, my family has been exceptionally supportive. Tom, my husband, sacrificed most. He patiently allowed me to be married to this project for as long as it took to do it right, which went on far longer than I originally expected. My sister gave constant encouragement over a very long haul and an incredibly committed eagle eye in reviewing the final draft. My mother, father, aunt, children, and grandchildren also lost much of my time and attention during this gestation period, as did other relatives and good friends. Yet all of them continuously expressed support. Without that, the experience would have been much different, and the end product would have suffered.

I also relied heavily on family, friends, and personal and professional acquaintances for honest feedback and suggestions for improvement at every stage of the development process. They all came through with invaluable assistance. I especially thank the following people for reading the entire manuscript, giving detailed comments from a consumer perspective, and in some cases providing material for the book: Gwen and Don Brock, Beth Freeland, Robert Forte, Beth Graham, Briana Burns, Janet Bias, and Stephanie Arthur. Nick Nortelli and Linda Holsonback both gave me incredibly useful comments based on their professional experiences in healthcare, and both were extremely helpful in other ways as well. Vicki Rosen, my favorite librarian, not only reviewed the manuscript, giving detailed comments, but also gave me much research assistance.

The medical and healthcare industry facts I used in the book were also reviewed by several experts. Pat Salber, MD, was so generous with her time and assistance that I truly do not believe I could have made this book into what I wanted it to be without her help. Kevin Fickenscher, MD, was extremely generous in allowing me to use some of his material to illustrate the concepts in Chapter 16. Steve Shortell, Dean of the School of Public Health at the University of California at Berkeley, reviewed the draft in its entirety and gave some key recommendations for improvement. Ken Covinsky, MD, Director of The VA National Quality Scholars Fellowship Program, was good enough to coordinate assistance from physician participants in that program to review several example stories used in the book. I am truly appreciative of the time, attention, and expert feedback these physicians gave toward making these stories accurate medically and appropriate in their advice to consumers. Any inaccuracies or poor advice remaining in the stories are, of course, my own responsibility, but I incorporated their excellent suggestions as much as I understood them. The participating physicians were doctors Jayna Holroyd-Leduc, Mike Steinman, Kenneth Chuang, Liz Burton, Edgar Pierluissi, and Serge Lindner.

Daniel Pound, MD, and Dave Thom, MD, at the University of California at San Francisco Medical Center, also gave me their valuable advice and assistance, as did Michelle Caughey, MD, with Kaiser Permanente. Julie Haugen, medical librarian for the University of California at San Francisco, gave me excellent suggestions for trustworthy website references, including steering me to the work and website of the Medical Librarians Association. Hazel Keimowitz, Manager, Prevention Programs at the Office of Health Care Information at the federal Agency for Healthcare Research and Quality, read my chapter on clinical prevention and gave good suggestions for improvement. Lisa Joyner at the National Committee for Quality Assurance gave freely of her time under difficult circumstances to make sure I got appropriate information to pass on to consumers.

Mike Phillips at Willis Insurance Services read an early draft and gave me thought-provoking comments. Paulette Wrede, Benefits Manager at Levi Strauss, gave me helpful thoughts on the concept of the book early on. Angie Espinoza, Benefits Manager for the Archdiocese of San Francisco, read the manuscript and gave very useful feedback from a human resources and consumer perspective. Roger Arlen of The Arlen Group believed in the message of this book enough that he built it into his employee benefits consulting business.

During the long period of writing, I had lots of good editorial help. Early on, Laurie Masters gave it her all. John Renesch served as developmental editor and terrific coach in the initial stages. Susan Tasaki contributed her experience, sound judgment, and editorial review toward the end. For the final brutal but exhilarating round, Brookes Nohlgren came through with flying colors as both copy and developmental editor. Ellen Reid, book shepherd extraordinaire, coordinated the professional support team that ultimately brought the book to life in a wonderfully creative process. Laren Bright, a very special wordsmith, was part of that team, as was Jack Barnard, who taught me how to hone my message for vibrant clarity. Pam Terry, my book designer, did awesome work.

I am exceptionally grateful to Roberta Ryan, who not only gave me heartening encouragement and feedback on the manuscript but who also put me in touch with Peter Winter, whose cartoons transform the book into a much more readable package than it would have been without them. But Peter gave me more than just the support of his cartoons. With his warm, radiant wisdom he also gave me cheering on at some of the times I most needed it.

Many, many others helped in their own ways. Please know, all of you, that I am very appreciative of your support.

Table of Contents

Preface

During my more than 20 years as a healthcare administration professional, I watched many perplexed consumers try to navigate the healthcare maze. I have seen them wrestle with confusing terminology and complicated paperwork. I have heard the mounting frustration as people struggle to figure out what to do in the ever-changing healthcare landscape. My heart has always gone out to them, and I always tried to help each and every frustrated healthcare consumer I came across. Being part of the system, I understand much that most people don't. Finally, as a way to help more consumers, I decided to write this book. To be free of any bias I might have or be seen to have if I continued to represent any particular healthcare provider or health plan while writing the book, I left my employment inside the industry. I am now an employee benefits consultant. This puts me in a related field but no longer directly representing medical care or health insurance.

Two particular events had significant impact on what I decided to include in the book.

The first event was that I was shocked to find out the extent of the quality problems in U.S. healthcare. This shock came as I was doing research for the book. After all my years working in the industry, I was not aware that gaps in medical quality in the U.S. are as extensive as they are. I discovered that the data about the astounding gaps in quality has been carefully verified but relatively poorly publicized. This is a symptom of how embarrassing this issue is to the medical community. There are many physicians and other medical professionals who are still in denial about this major problem. I, like most healthcare professionals, had known only about what was happening immediately around me, in my own health plan. The plan I worked for measured many aspects of the quality of care it provided and did well in the measurements. I was blown away by the data showing how poorly the medical industry was doing across the country. When I fully realized the extent of the problem, I knew that consumers needed to be alerted to it and told how to protect themselves. This became the major focus of the book.

At about the same time that I discovered the data on the huge quality gaps in U.S. healthcare, one of my closest relatives became a victim of this very problem. She became seriously and permanently disabled as the result of not getting appropriate medical care. This made me very angry. I vowed to use her experience to teach as many other people as possible how to avoid the hidden pitfalls of the healthcare system.

There are two key things I have worked hard to accomplish for you, the reader, in this book. First, I spent special effort to be accurate and to gather the most important information for you. I did my own extensive research and then asked medical and public health experts on quality to review my writing. Second, because I know the information is complex, I have split it out into what I hope are digestible "chunks" that will make sense separately and that combined will give you a sense of the whole. As I wrote, I asked many average consumers to read the drafts and give me feedback about what made sense to them and what did not. Their reviews were extremely valuable in shaping the finished book.

So, you can see that this book was written to be as consumer-friendly as possible. It is not and is not intended to be an academic analysis of the issues. Therefore, it is different from many books written on this topic. If you are looking for an academic and scholarly tome, this is not the book for you. Though the information presented is quite accurate, the analysis has purposely been kept at a high overview level, presented in consumer-oriented terms.

> *Poor Huck was too distressed to smile, but the old man laughed loud and joyously, shook up the details of his anatomy from head to foot, and ended by saying that such a laugh was money in a man's pocket, because it cut down the doctor's bills like everything.*
> —Mark Twain, from *Tom Sawyer*

I know from the "test" consumers who have read drafts of this book that complex healthcare information is dry reading no matter how much effort is put into making it more readable. To keep your journey through the book as fun as possible, I've included cartoons created by Peter Winter. Peter's skill at bringing us laughter through his pictures is a gift that will cut down on all of our doctor bills.

I truly hope this book works for you.

Introduction

The Institute of Medicine is a highly respected federal agency, part of the National Institutes of Health. The Institute's reports *To Err is Human,*[1] published in 2000, and *Crossing the Quality Chasm,*[2] published in 2001, describe the devastating gaps in quality in U.S. medical care. The reports are landmarks in American medicine that have alerted many within the healthcare industry to the extent of the quality crisis. *Crossing the Quality Chasm* identified the following goals for any healthcare system: Care should be Safe, Effective, Efficient, Personalized, Timely, and Equitable. Far too often today's U.S. healthcare does not reach these goals, even when we pay dearly for it.

The U.S. healthcare system is overwhelmingly complex. For many consumers, trying to get good medical care can feel like traveling a bewildering maze full of decision points. Keeping track of healthcare system changes to make sure you don't pay too much or miss out on something you're entitled to can be tedious and time-consuming. Getting through the system at all is challenging enough—making sure that the care you receive is of high quality can be even more difficult.

The process has become so complicated that it almost seems as if there is a plot to make getting good healthcare as baffling and frustrating as possible for the patient. And while most of us would like to go down the road to quality medical care with the confidence of a savvy consumer, we often find ourselves frustrated, stuck in a system we need, and powerless to navigate a baffling and constantly changing terrain.

Without a proper road map, many people just close their eyes to make healthcare decisions, hoping that any mistakes won't be too costly. Their quest for good healthcare is haphazard at best.

The perplexity is enough to make an ordinary person want to give up.

Placing Blame

I don't need to convince anyone that the situation has reached crisis level. No one is happy with the current system, not even healthcare providers. Those who pay for healthcare are outraged at skyrocketing costs. Providers claim they are not being paid enough. There are increasing claims about poor quality. The complexities of the options and rules for getting care are increasing. Yet, there are no clear villains to blame—not doctors, not hospitals, not insurance companies, not government. All players in the healthcare "game," including consumers, have had a part in creating the current crisis.

Many of the players have contributed unknowingly and through little or no fault of their own. Employers, who pay the largest chunk of healthcare costs, choose healthcare plans largely based on cost rather than quality. The major reason is simple: In order to remain profitable in an increasingly competitive world market, they have to watch the bottom line at all times. And, like consumers, most employers don't know how to define healthcare quality, so are unable to distinguish among health plan choices. In turn, under pressure from the employers to contain costs, many health plans and insurance companies prioritize costs over quality. In addition, they have their own cost increase pressures in providing care to members. Convoluted payment mechanisms between employers, consumers, insurance companies, and providers have caused health plans to create convoluted rules and systems for providing care.

Doctors and hospitals have increased their prices. They have increasing costs of their own. With regard to quality, most physician and hospital payment mechanisms have no built-in incentives to reward high quality or quality improvement. As a result, relatively few physicians and hospitals have made it a priority to improve the quality of care they provide, even as they increase their prices.

Consumers have rebelled against restrictions in their choice of providers, resenting loss of flexibility and thinking the restrictions decrease quality. Thus consumers unknowingly cause an increase in costs while possibly decreasing the value of the healthcare they get. In general, the more choices of providers a consumer has in a health plan, the less control the health plan has over quality or costs. (This will be explained as you read on.)

As you can see, it's difficult to place blame for the system's complexity, inefficiency, inconsistent quality, and skyrocketing costs squarely and solely on any party or practice.

Getting the Best Care You Can

Although there are many problems in the U.S. healthcare system, the major focus of this book is on healthcare quality. Strong evidence indicates that most people in the U.S. are not getting the best care as often as they should. There is a huge

> Strong evidence indicates that most people in the U.S. are not getting the best care as often as they should.

gap between the quality of average medical care in the U.S. and the quality of the best care that we know is available from some providers.

How This Book Can Help You

In order to confidently take action to improve your health and healthcare, you must be armed with the facts and be clear about what you want. I have written *Surviving Healthcare* to give you those advantages.

Although this book can't eliminate the hazards of today's medical system, it can serve as a compass, steadily pointing you in the direction of your goal. As we survey the problems and challenges of the healthcare system together, you will find yourself increasingly able to distinguish poor or mediocre care from superior medical practices. This book will shed light in dark corners of myth and misinformation and guide you toward a more complete understanding of the issues.

Notes to the Reader

Before we go further, I've included here some suggestions on how you might approach this book, depending on your particular situation.

How to Approach This Book

If you are well: If you don't currently have any pain, disability, or apparent disease, you'd probably rather not think too much about healthcare. But please remember, it's never too early to prepare for your health future. To live a long, healthy life as free as possible from disability, you need to figure out your biggest personal health risks and how to avoid them as best you can. To do this, follow these steps:

1. Find out which preventive healthcare services you need, based on your age, sex, and personal health risks (see Chapter 7).

2. Bone up on even better ways to stay healthy through preventive *self*-care (see Chapter 8).

3. Be prepared to get the best help when you need it.

   Look over Chapters 9 through 16 to see what high-quality care looks like, so you will know what to ask for in the future. Then put this book where you can refer to it when you need it.

   When the time comes for you to choose among the many health plan options (see Chapters 17 through 22), to explore alternatives to standard medical treatment (see Chapter 24), or to figure out how to get the best care for a specific diagnosis (see Appendix A), this book will help you.

If you are ill: Read this book from start to finish. Every chapter will help you. Concentrate especially on Chapters 9 through 16 to find out what high-quality healthcare looks like.

If your health challenges require the services of many different facilities and providers, you'll want to study about Coordinated Care (Chapter 12) in particular, since the degree to which your care is effectively coordinated will be crucial to the quality of healthcare you receive.

The Appendices of this book (Part VII) are full of additional information to help you find high-quality, reliable medical information tailored to your particular interests and needs.

Other Factors That Will Influence You

Various factors will influence how you use medical care and how you choose health insurance coverage. They will therefore also influence how you use this book. These include:

- Your age.
- Your personal health risk factors.
- The region of the country you live in.
- Whether you are male or female.
- Your race.
- Your sexual orientation.
- Your income bracket.
- Whether you are single or married.
- Whether or not you have children.
- Whether you live in a rural or an urban area.
- The healthcare coverage options available to you, possibly offered by your employer and/or your spouse's employer.

If, for example, you are a typical 26-year-old single female living in Los Angeles, you likely have few health problems and don't want to spend much time thinking about healthcare. Your best use of this book would be to skim the entire book, then go back and concentrate on prevention (Chapters 7 and 8) to help you define your long-term health risks and how you can plan your life and medical care to decrease those risks.

Starting early to decrease risk is the absolute best approach. Because you live in an urban area that has been well studied, you will find some good resources listed in the Appendices to rate the quality of many local medical groups, hospitals, and health plans. Depending on which health plans your employer offers (assuming you are employed and have health benefits), you may have a high-quality, lower-cost health plan available that could serve you well.

If, however, you are a 46-year-old male living in a rural area that has relatively few doctors and hospitals, your situation is quite different. First, your age suggests you need to quickly assess your personal disease risk factors. You determine your disease risks by working with your doctor to assess your family health history, your health history and current state of health, and your lifestyle factors. I recommend that you read this entire book carefully, especially the information on prevention (Chapters 7 and 8).

Living in a rural area, you are less likely to find sources of quality comparison data on your local doctors and hospitals. This means that you need to understand the elements of quality well so that you can assess your local providers and encourage quality improvement if necessary. Living in a rural area also means that you are less likely to have health benefits through your employer, because people in rural areas are often either self-employed or work for very small employers. You may have a choice of individual coverage plans. Because your choice of providers is likely limited to those few available locally, your choice of health insurance plans may not be based on which providers are on a plan's list.

You can see in these examples that you will need to assess your own particular situation to determine how to use this book. Some parts of the book apply to everyone. Other parts are more applicable to some people than to others. I have done my best to include enough information so that each of you, whatever your situation, can use this book to find better healthcare and achieve greater health.

PART I

THE HEALTHCARE LANDSCAPE

Chapter 1
You Are Here: The Sad Condition of Today's Healthcare

Chapter 2
Where We'd Like to Be: Defining Ideal Healthcare

Chapter 3
Getting There

Part I will help orient you to the obstacles you'll face in your pursuit of the best possible healthcare. Knowing where you are starting, where you are headed, and what some of your obstacles will be along the way will help prepare you to reach your goal.

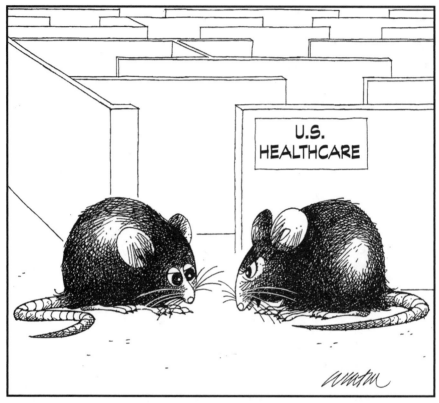

"I'VE BEEN ASKED TO RUN SOME SENSELESS MAZES IN MY TIME, BUT THIS TAKES THE CAKE."

Flora

When she was young, Flora was a pretty, vivacious, charming brunette. She always looked much younger than her age, and she anticipated living a long and active life, just as her mother had. Flora's mother lived to be 95, and was vital and happy right up to the end.

Flora's life didn't turn out that way—and it very possibly could have if she had made different choices about her healthcare. Now in her mid–80s, Flora lives in pain and misery much of the time. She is 90% blind, suffers from severe osteoporosis, and never leaves her house more than a couple of hours at a time because she doesn't have the strength to handle more than that.

Flora had volunteered quite a lot of time to a local medical charity when she was younger. She worked with the medical community and knew which doctors were considered to be the best in her town. Rather than join an HMO, where she would not be able to use these "best" doctors, she maintained a PPO insurance plan. With such a plan she was never required to choose a primary-care doctor, and not having someone coordinating her medical care ultimately resulted in her poor health in later life.

Flora's blindness is due to glaucoma, a common disorder that increases in frequency with advancing age and is generally without symptoms before vision is affected. The tragedy is that it could easily have been prevented had Flora gotten regular eye examinations. But no one recommended this course to her because Flora chose to see only specialists as needed for specific illnesses. She thought this was the way to get the highest quality care.

At one point she saw a cardiologist for a mild heart murmur. She developed a good relationship with him, and from then on considered him to be in effect her primary-care doctor. But he did not look at the overall picture of her health.

When she finally developed severe back pain from vertebral spine fractures caused by osteoporosis, her cardiologist referred her to an orthopedic surgeon. By then the disease was fairly advanced. The risk of developing osteoporosis could have been greatly reduced—if not completely eliminated—if she had taken calcium and vitamin D supplements and exercised regularly. But because of her mild heart murmur, her cardiologist told her not to exercise. (I have the same type of slight heart murmur, and I have exercised regularly for the last 20 years with the full blessing and encouragement of my doctors.)

Because of her blindness and severe osteoporosis, Flora now needs daily help at home with basic living needs like fixing meals. She is using up her life savings for this very expensive support, but she has no choice. She's terrified of what will happen to her when her savings are used up.

Flora feels betrayed by the healthcare system. Because she had inside connections to the system thanks to her extensive volunteer work in the medical community, she thought she had a better-than-average understanding of how to get the best care. But none of the many healthcare specialists she worked with gave her the advice she needed to prevent the disabilities she now suffers.

1 You Are Here: The Sad Condition of Today's Healthcare

Education is what you get when you read the fine print. Experience is what you get when you don't.   —Anonymous

In This Chapter...
Grim news and startling statistics about where we are and how far we have to go.

To begin the journey towards high-quality healthcare, the first thing we must do is to understand where we are starting. Much of the news isn't good.

The sad, scary, true story about Flora on the previous pages illustrates how our healthcare system often betrays our trust. One major problem is that people are able to seek only specialist care. This can result in fragmented personal care. The story also illustrates that not all physicians give the best advice or treatment. In Flora's case, her cardiologist fortunately never actually gave her bad care. He simply did not look out for her in the best way. He should have strongly advised her to have a primary-care doctor who could ensure she got the basic preventive screening tests she should have had. And, rather than tell her she should not exercise, he should have worked with her to design an exercise program that would be appropriate for her heart condition and that would promote her health in other ways.

Though Flora's medical care was never outrageously wrong, as does happen in some cases, it nevertheless had very tragic results. Care of questionable thoroughness and effectiveness combined with lack of coordination leads to unnecessary illness, disability, and premature death more often than most consumers realize. Actual errors in care add even more to the total picture of poor quality in U.S. healthcare. Treatment that does not meet the highest standards of quality is provided far too often, as statistics cited below will show.

> The Institute of Medicine has indicated that as many as 98,000 people die from medical errors in a given year.

Startling Statistics About Medical Errors and Poor Quality

The truth gets uglier still. The following statistics are shocking and disturbing to most people. They reflect the seriousness of our current crisis.

- The Institute of Medicine has indicated that as many as 98,000 people die from medical errors in a given year. That's more than the total who die from motor vehicle accidents, breast cancer, and AIDS combined.[1]

Many deaths could be prevented if hospitals had better quality-control systems.

- In addition to downright errors, other types of quality gaps in hospitals as well as other parts of U.S. healthcare cause an additional 57,000 avoidable deaths each year. These are deaths of people with health insurance and good access to healthcare.[2]

- On average across the country, patients receive only 55% of recommended care (care based on the latest scientific evidence of what works best). This includes preventive care, acute care, and care for chronic (long-term) illnesses.[3]

- 20% of patients with chronic conditions receive the wrong care.[4]

- An estimated 50% of premature deaths from nine key diseases could be prevented.[5]

- 30% of U.S. healthcare dollars are wasted due to overuse, underuse, or misuse of medical care and to administrative inefficiency.[6]

- Hospital-acquired infections are a leading cause of death in the United States.[7] Postoperative bloodstream infections alone are estimated to have killed more than 3,000 people in the year 2000, or resulted in hospital stays on average 11 days longer than normal and with added average costs of $57,727 per case. Postoperative reopening of surgical incisions resulted in additional deaths, an average of 9.4 additional hospital days, and $40,000 in additional costs per case. These are only 2 of the 18 hospital-acquired causes of death, excess length of stay, and added costs.[8] Many deaths could be prevented if hospitals had better quality-control systems.

- More than 770,000 people are injured or die from medication errors in U.S. hospitals every year (known in the industry as adverse drug events, or ADEs). These errors include giving the wrong dose (either too much, too little, too often, or not often enough), giving a drug to a patient known to be allergic to that drug, giving a drug to the wrong patient, and others. Most medication errors do not cause injury, but the statistics shown here prove that far too many do.[9]

Other Signposts Marking What's Happening in Healthcare

Here are some other signposts that indicate the crisis in today's healthcare system.

Waning Consumer Confidence

With all the news stories about people being victimized by their health plans, especially HMOs, most consumers are very uneasy about being able to get the care they need if they become ill.

Skyrocketing Costs

The costs of healthcare are increasing at an alarming rate, and some say they will double in the next five years. Unable to absorb these increases and remain competitive, many employers are passing on the additional costs to employees in the form of increased premiums, copayments, coinsurance, and deductibles. Worse, these higher costs are not always yielding higher-quality healthcare or better overall health.

Ever-Changing Affiliations

Keeping track of which physicians are on a plan's list at any given time is becoming increasingly challenging and time-consuming for consumers and even for the plans themselves. Many doctors are opting out of their contracts, which is leaving fewer in-network doctors to choose from and forcing patients to leave behind established relationships to seek new doctors from an approved list. Also, health plan contracts with hospitals, laboratories, and other service providers are constantly changing, thus adding to consumers' confusion, frustration, and fear that they won't get the help they need at critical times.

Baffling Prescription Management

Prescription drug coverage is often separate from medical care coverage, with no connection between the physician who prescribes the drug and the company that determines which drugs are covered under a health plan and the amount of the copayment. With the advent of multi-tier drug copayments,[10] figuring out what a prescribed drug will actually cost the consumer out-of-pocket has become even more confusing.

> The goal of finding quality healthcare today is an achievable goal.

All in all, the road ahead looks pretty grim for the average consumer: constantly rising confusion, growing frustration, and escalating out-of-pocket costs with no apparent increase in quality.

The Good News

There is some good news, however: The U.S. offers some of the world's best healthcare, although this is effectively inaccessible to consumers who don't know what to look for. The goal of finding quality healthcare today is an achievable goal. All you have to do is become a savvy consumer. The information in this book will help you increase your odds of finding, rather than happening upon, the high-quality care you deserve.

Betty

Betty is a charming woman in her mid-80s. Much like Flora, whose story introduced Chapter 1, Betty was a pretty brunette, very energetic, and vivacious in her youth.

Unlike Flora, though, Betty still has much of her old spunk. She lives alone with no daily help, loves to cook for her family, still drives, and relishes her independence. Though she is slower at most things than she once was, she feels pretty good most of the time, with only occasional aches and pains. She has a very full social life with her family and friends and attends many church functions.

How could these two lives become so very different?

The reason for the difference is that Betty has gotten excellent, thorough medical care over the last 30 years. Twenty-five years ago, she was diagnosed with cancer. Fortunately, it was caught at an early stage, treated appropriately and has been in remission ever since. Her doctors have made sure she received all of the best preventive care and screening for other types of cancer and other diseases as well as the most effective treatments for the acute illnesses she has occasionally had. As part of her preventive care, her primary-care doctor encourages her to keep up her regular exercise, even though it is more difficult for her to walk now that her osteoarthritis is getting a bit worse as she ages. With the overview of her whole health picture, her doctor is able to weigh the benefits against the difficulties and advise her as to what is best for her, overall.

2 Where We'd Like to Be: Defining Ideal Healthcare

Knowledge is power.
—Sir Francis Bacon

In This Chapter...
The destination is better healthcare and, more importantly, excellent health.

Betty is very lucky. Neither she nor Flora had good information to help them find high-quality healthcare. In fact, Flora paid top dollar to go to the doctors she thought would give her the best health results, but she did not get what she paid for. Betty, on the other hand, chose to join and stay with an HMO that was more affordable than her other options. She happened to get a bargain. Betty's care was thorough and coordinated and incorporated the best treatments. Flora's care was not thorough or well coordinated, and it may or may not have incorporated the best medical treatments. The point is that unless you know exactly what to look for, the quality of the care you get will be based on pure luck.

These stories are not about the difference in quality between PPOs and HMOs. In fact, you can get excellent quality care in PPOs, HMOs, POS plans, EPOs, or essentially any type of health plan. But to maximize your chances of getting high-quality care, you need to know what the real thing looks like.

As with any of life's journeys, in our search for high-quality healthcare we won't know where to start—and we're unlikely to get anywhere (unless by pure luck)—unless we know where we want to end up.

What We Want for Ourselves

Ask the majority of Americans what they want out of their healthcare system and they will say the following:

• To know I am getting the best care possible.

- To know that my doctor knows and will always tell me what I need to do to prevent/delay/decrease the severity of any major illness I might be vulnerable to.

- To know that my doctor knows exactly what my current problem is, what has caused it, and how best to cure it without any serious side effects.

- To know that my doctor can treat me as soon as possible when I have a problem, at a cost I can afford, and with great respect for me, my time, and my lifestyle.

High-quality healthcare is what we all deserve.

- To trust my doctor to work in respectful partnership with me in making decisions about my care.

- To know that any care I receive from any part of the healthcare system is well coordinated with all the other care I receive or might receive in the future.

- To spend my limited financial resources only on necessary, effective, and reasonably priced healthcare services.

Many of us, especially if we have not had much interaction with the healthcare system, assume or hope that we will get everything we need when we need it. But the fact is that, with today's healthcare system, we rarely get all of the aspects of good care listed above. In fact, as stated before, the situation is worse than the vast majority of consumers know about.

Having said that, the forecast isn't all gloom and doom. If you browse the websites listed in the Appendices, you will find that some players in our nation's healthcare industry are working diligently to make things better.

Many of these efforts are still in conceptual stages, but keep in mind that envisioning improvement is a major step in making it happen. Every great achievement of humanity had its humble beginnings as a concept in the mind of one or more forward-looking people. You can do your part, too, by insisting on high quality in all of your medical care.

Know What to Look For

Everyone has some notion of what high-quality healthcare is. Following are some of the criteria many people associate with high-quality healthcare:

- Doctors who will spend time to answer all questions and who will get to the heart of all medical concerns.

- Doctors who help prevent illness and detect and treat all medical problems at an early stage.

- Convenient access, choice of physician, and low out-of-pocket expenses.

- "Cosmetic" factors such as the quality of waiting room amenities and the friendliness of receptionists.

In fact, high-quality healthcare incorporates most (but not all) of these factors as well as many others not mentioned here. Healthcare services that combine top-notch clinical quality, respect for the full human person, convenience, and affordability are not widely available. Some facilities and providers offer more of these elements than others do, and finding the superior facilities can often be a quest.

High-quality healthcare is what we all deserve. Betty's real-life example shows us the quality of care we should be getting. Unfortunately, most of us, like Flora, don't get this level of care. The bottom line is that we simply can't be sure of getting it unless we take charge and find it.

This book will help you do just that. It will explain the following factors that comprise high-quality healthcare. You should become familiar with these factors and know how to look for them in your own care to make sure you're getting the best.

- **Prevention.** This is the most important factor of all. Many people don't get thorough advice and care for preventing illness, and this puts them in jeopardy of dying prematurely or becoming disabled unnecessarily.

- **Measuring the Quality of Care.** If your doctor and hospital don't measure the quality of the care they provide, they don't know how they measure up. If they do assess their own level of quality but don't release that information publicly, YOU will not know how they measure up.

- **Getting the Most Effective Treatments.** Medical research has proven that certain treatments are the most effective for specific diagnoses. However, many doctors are not providing these proven treatments. You will find out how to make sure you get the best treatments.

- **Avoiding Medical Mistakes.** In addition to the problem of not prescribing scientifically proven treatments, many doctors and other care providers inadvertently make mistakes in giving care to patients. You will discover the alarming extent of these problems and how to best protect yourself against them.

- **Coordination of Care.** Our current U.S. healthcare system is highly uncoordinated. Especially if you are seriously ill, this can cause you to receive very poor-quality care. If you have multiple doctors, for example, each will most likely not know what the others are doing. Or the emergency room where you wind up unconscious will not know the drugs you are allergic to or the serious medical problems you have. You will learn what to look for in coordinated care and how to coordinate your care if that is not being done for you.

- **Patient-Centered Care.** The most effective healthcare treats each patient with respect as a full human being and takes into account the wide diversity among us. Respect includes making healthcare services convenient for the patient to use as well as making sure the patient participates as a partner in making decisions about his or her own care.

- **The Pros and Cons of Managed Care.** The management of care can contribute greatly to improving quality of care. You will learn which aspects of managed care benefit consumers and which do not.

- **Integrated Care Systems.** The highest-quality medical care is provided in systems that pull all parts of care together in a manner that is organized, efficient, and effective *for the patient*. This type of care is hard but not impossible to find in American medicine. You must know what to look for.

- **Information Technology.** Electronic information and communication systems have revolutionized modern life. One way this has happened is that a vast amount of information is easily accessible to all of us through the Internet. Healthcare consumers can benefit from this by getting good data to help steer them to high-quality medical providers and the best treatments. Another way electronics have transformed our lives is to enhance processes of work. The medical industry has been slow to adopt Information Technology as a tool to assist in improving quality of care, but some providers are more up-to-speed than others, and new uses of this technology are being implemented every day. We will soon see big changes in medical care as a result. Savvy consumers will know how to use the Internet wisely to improve their chances of getting the best healthcare, and they will know what to look for in finding providers who best use technology to improve care.

Keep this list in mind as you continue to read. Throughout the book, you will see time and time again the importance of consumers learning to distinguish high-quality healthcare from poor-quality care and taking on the responsibility for making sure they get the best.

3 Getting There

Do not follow where the path may lead. Go instead where there is no path and leave a trail.　　　　　　　　　—Ralph Waldo Emerson

---

In This Chapter...

• The methods used to improve quality in the Japanese auto industry can be and in some cases are being applied to U.S. healthcare.

• There are steps you can take to get better healthcare now.

A Model for Improving Today's Healthcare System

In the 1950s, the phrase "made in Japan" brought to mind images of cheap, low-quality, unreliable products. In a determined attempt to revitalize their postwar economy, Japanese manufacturers set out to develop reliable methods for massively improving the quality of their products.

The Japanese auto industry, in particular, took on the challenge of competing with U.S. automakers so successfully that they took Detroit by surprise and compelled them to take notice. As a result, U.S. automakers were forced to improve their processes, offer longer guarantees, and match the reliability and quality of their Japanese counterparts. Eventually, in fact, several U.S. industries embraced Japanese quality-improvement techniques.

Our healthcare system, unfortunately, has no equivalent competitor, foreign or domestic, to spur its improvement. That leaves only us, the consumers, to urge needed changes. Just as American car buyers became discontented with the mediocre products Detroit had to offer and compelled the industry to change its ways, healthcare consumers must become catalysts for changing our medical system.

TQM

The body of knowledge and practices the Japanese used to revolutionize the quality of their products and services is called Total Quality Management, or TQM. Its emphasis on continuous improvement can be broadly applied to any industry. In fact, TQM has already been used extensively in various organizations within the healthcare industry. Some have been more successful than others at improving their medical care processes. Those projects whose goals have not been clearly consumer-oriented have had limited success. I believe that if TQM were applied as it was intended by its creators, the American management consultants Drs. W. E. Deming and J. M. Juran, TQM could help change the healthcare industry in the ways it needs to be changed. Those U.S. healthcare organizations that are successfully improving their processes using TQM or other quality enhancement tools offer an excellent example for others in the industry to follow.

Let's look at five key TQM principles. I've included a brief example of how Japanese auto manufacturers implemented each as well as some thoughts on how the U.S. healthcare system could adopt them. You might think of the resulting effort as Total Healthcare Quality Management (THQM).

1. Customers Come First.

The product should meet customer needs and desires, not the needs and desires of the producers of the product. In the auto industry, this meant, for example, coming up with innovative ways to improve gas mileage. Japanese auto engineers figured this out much sooner than their American counterparts.

How this applies to U.S. healthcare: Insist that your healthcare providers focus primarily on *your* needs, not the needs of the physician or the hospital or the lab, in providing your care. For example, care providers should make it easy for you to get all your questions answered.

2. Focus on Strong Leadership for Quality.

All leaders of the organization must continuously and strongly demonstrate their commitment to improving the quality of the product. Upper management at Toyota led the company's quality-improvement efforts. The results they helped Toyota achieve prove the value of leadership for quality improvement.

How this applies to U.S. healthcare: Your doctor, the president of your doctor's medical group, the CEO of your chosen hospital, and anyone else in a leadership position in relation to your healthcare should demonstrate his or her commitment to improving and maintaining the quality of the care you receive. You should be able to see evidence of a commitment to high-quality healthcare, once you know what to look for.

Ask your doctor, your hospital, and your health plan if they participate in any unbiased, third-party measurements of the level of quality they provide compared to that of competitors. If they do not participate in any third-party measurement programs, tell them you believe they should. Also ask them for information on any internal quality measurement and improvement programs they currently have, and exactly what improvements have been made through these programs. Do the results show actual improvements in outcomes of patient care? Get the details. Don't just accept blanket statements that the doctor/hospital/health plan is "committed to the highest quality." If the proof isn't there, it may mean that the leaders of the organizations providing your care are not too concerned about the level of quality they provide.

Informed consumers can cause positive change.

3. Processes Are Key.

Process improvement means focusing on enhancing the outcomes of every step of the process of producing the product or service. For example, this would include increasing the on-time delivery of parts in a manufacturing process, decreasing the time on hold for customers at call centers, decreasing order process time, decreasing inventory storage costs, and so on. To improve quality, Japanese auto manufacturers scrutinized every detail of their manufacturing processes, such as whether to install the steering wheel before the dashboard—or vice-versa. They found that improving work processes yielded higher-quality results than did hiring or training better workers or obtaining better equipment.

How this applies to U.S. healthcare: Some care providers have developed better coordinated, more effective, more efficient ways to deliver the healthcare services you need. Many others have not made these improvements. See Chapters 9 through 16 to understand what you should look for and ask for.

4. Get the Facts.

Gather accurate, complete facts about current practices before deciding how to improve. The Japanese had to assess exactly how poorly their cars stood up to U.S. products before they could plan their improvement efforts.

How this applies to U.S. healthcare: Many studies have confirmed that U.S. doctors vary widely in their understanding and use of the latest medical knowledge. Most doctors have not invested in measuring how well their care stacks up against that of other physicians or against the best possible care. Search out and use healthcare providers who can show evidence of the quality of their care. See Appendix B for a list of quality comparison resources.

5. Work in Teams.

Teamwork pays off in improved quality. Japanese automakers took this concept to its ultimate, including all levels of employees in quality-improvement projects. They included factory workers in project teams assigned to solve manufacturing problems. The factory workers, the ones who actually did the work and intimately knew the manufacturing processes, came up with creative and effective solutions.

How this applies to U.S. healthcare: You will get the best medical care from providers who work well in teams. Find a doctor who proactively and genuinely collaborates with and learns from the other players on the healthcare team—nurses, receptionists, nutritionists, other doctors, physical therapists, lab techs, pharmacists, surgeons, and so forth. All of these parties should be working together to ensure that you are taken care of properly. See Chapters 12 and 15 for details.

As you read through the following chapters, you will see how these TQM principles, if properly applied, could improve U.S. healthcare.

What You Can Do to Improve Your Healthcare

Informed consumers can cause positive change. Power in any consumer-based system lies with the customer, even in a system as impersonal and entrenched as U.S. healthcare. The greatest way for you to improve your health and ultimately change the medical system is by taking charge of your own healthcare and making your voice heard. What does that mean?

Accept Nothing Less Than Excellence

By selecting only quality health plans, choosing doctors and hospitals with proven (measurable) track records for high quality, and insisting on working with their doctors to get the best care, healthcare consumers cause improvements in the system. Mediocre healthcare can only exist when customers are uninformed, apathetic, or resigned to accepting care of undetermined quality.

Help Your Providers Do Their Best

Locating a high-quality provider is not enough. You must vigilantly work with your doctors and other providers to make sure you get the best possible care on an ongoing basis.

(To find out exactly what this means, see Part III and Part IV). By becoming more involved in your healthcare treatment, you engage the doctor to become more involved, and thus improve the care you receive.

How can you accomplish these things?

1. Discover the truth about many healthcare myths people have that interfere with their getting the best care. (Chapter 4)

2. Find out how to choose a good doctor and health plan. (Chapter 5)

3. Learn how to take a partnering role with your doctor. (Chapters 6 and 13)

4. Discover the proven, amazingly high value of prevention and what it can do for you. (Chapters 7 and 8)

5. Learn what high-quality care looks like so you can demand it and know when you are and are not getting it. (Chapters 9 through 16)

6. Find out why higher cost doesn't always mean higher quality. (Chapter 23)

The Key to Your Health

The most important message I have for you is that **you must take charge of your own health and healthcare.** You will need to seek high-quality care in ways few consumers know how to do.

To maximize your health, you must take full responsibility for it. This means your lifestyle as well as your healthcare. There are two reasons for this.

1. No amount of medical care can substitute for living a healthful lifestyle. Research shows that personal/lifestyle behavior forms 50% of the basis of our state of health, while medical care accounts for only 10%, on average.[1] Specifically, not smoking, keeping your weight at an appropriate level, getting regular exercise, and eating a healthy, high-fiber diet rich in vegetables, fruits, and whole grains—and maintaining these practices over your entire life—can do far more to keep you healthy than any medical care (see Chapters 7 and 8).

2. When you *do* require medical services, you'll want to be familiar with what high-quality care looks like. You may not get the best care unless you know what to ask for.

Nobody but you can make that happen. (See Chapters 9 through 16 for in-depth discussions of high-quality care.)

PART II

GETTING ON TRACK TO
HIGHER-QUALITY HEALTHCARE

Chapter 4
Myths and the Mess They Make

Chapter 5
All Doctors and Health Plans Are Not Created Equal

Chapter 6
Your Role in Getting High-Quality Healthcare

In Part II you will find information that is the starting point of your becoming a savvy healthcare consumer. You will discover the truth about common healthcare myths. Then you will find guidelines for the best ways to choose a physician and health plan. Following that you will find guidance on how to work with your doctor, your hospital, and other care providers to get the best care.

Think Differently

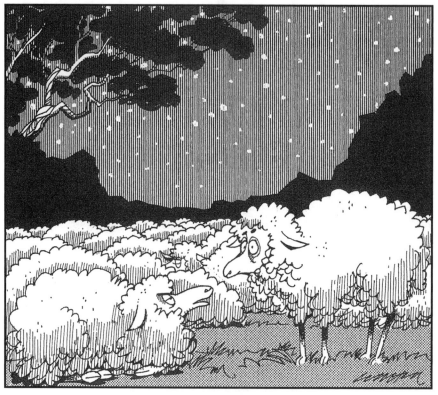

"TRY COUNTING SHEPHERDS"

4 Myths and the Mess They Make

That is what learning is. You suddenly understand something you've understood all your life, but in a new way. —Doris Lessing

In This Chapter...
- Why we need to think differently about healthcare.
- Eight important healthcare myths dispelled.

The next part of our journey leads us to examine what we think we know about healthcare. I've gathered eight commonly held, yet inaccurate, beliefs—myths—that lead many healthcare consumers away from their intended destination of excellent healthcare.

Myth-Perceptions

As healthcare consumers, we need to think differently about our role. After all, we are customers who have every right to demand better quality healthcare. We deserve that, but we need to do our part. To demand improvements for a better healthcare system in this country, and to receive better care, we need to learn more about the system. We can't improve something when we don't understand how it works. That's why it's important to address the following common misunderstandings before we go on.

Following each myth is a brief explanation about why it is not valid. You will find more information about most of these issues in later chapters.

Myth #1: "It's All the Insurance Companies' Fault"

Many consumers believe that health plans and insurance companies are responsible for the crisis in U.S. healthcare. The myth is: "If insurance companies and health plans would just get out of the way, leave doctors alone, and stop making things difficult, we would all get better healthcare."

This is far too simplistic. The insurance processes and payment mechanisms are not the only dysfunctional aspects of the system. That's like blaming teachers for all the faults in our educational system, or the police for all crime.

Our whole healthcare system is in crisis, and everyone involved shares responsibility for it. Everyone is at fault, including physicians, laboratories, medical equipment manufacturers, insurance agents, pharmacists, legislators, the courts, drug makers, hospitals, other healthcare professionals, consumers, and, of course, insurance companies and the health plans.

We are told that we have to pay high prices because of medical advances, yet much of the cost is due to poor organization as well as poor quality.

Physicians are key to our healthcare and although most are hardworking and dedicated to helping their patients, many U.S. physicians have been unable to keep pace with major advances in medical science. The result is that many outdated and/or unproven treatments are being provided, and there is wide variation in how physicians diagnose and treat any given set of symptoms. In addition, medical mistakes occur in alarming numbers, many of which go unreported.

And there are more problems. The medical care we receive is generally very poorly organized. Multiple doctors treating the same patient don't always communicate with one another. Information about emergency care received at a hospital often doesn't get to the patient's doctors. Patient calls to a health plan's call center often don't get to the patient's physician(s). And so on. As a result, the quality of care suffers.

This lack of organization of care is as much at fault in our healthcare crisis as is any group within the system. For example, patients with chronic kidney disease who are on kidney dialysis programs have far more contact with the healthcare system than do most people, yet there is clear evidence that these patients often do not receive preventive screening for other health risks.[1] One reason for this is poor coordination between the nephrologist (kidney specialist) and the patient's primary-care physician. The result is that the patient becomes more vulnerable to such risks as breast cancer, uterine cancer, prostate cancer, and diabetes-related problem detection and prevention.

Here's another example. If you wind up unconscious in an emergency room, the ER physician will, in most situations, have no way of knowing what medications you are on or are allergic to, even though this information may be well documented in your chart at your doctor's office. We accept this as just the way things are. To provide better care, every ER physician would need to be able to immediately access this type of information.

We are paying top dollar for medical care that is, in many cases, mediocre. When mediocre products and services are delivered to the consumer, and the consumer accepts such mediocrity, it suggests a major system failure—not simply an incidental glitch! We are told that we have to pay high prices because of medical advances, yet much of the cost is due to poor organization as well as poor quality. A disjointed system makes keeping our care semi-organized and roughly coordinated very costly. And while the direct cost in dollars is huge, the total cost also includes losses in life, quality of life, and productivity.

So, the fault is not just with the insurers and the plans. Many of our problems begin at the heart of where care is provided—in the doctors' offices and the hospitals.

Myth #2: "It's All About Money"

Another myth is that HMOs and other health plans impose controls on doctors and consumers solely for the purpose of saving money, without regard for and sometimes at the expense of quality. For example, restricting the choice of specialists often seems like a mechanism created simply to cut costs.

It is true that health plans vary in their commitment to high quality. It is also true that all health plans focus on cost controls to remain competitive. But what may not be obvious is that while some control mechanisms arise purely for reasons of cost, others have as a goal to promote higher quality. And some control mechanisms actually accomplish both.

For example, cost-control processes that also aid in coordinating care between primary-care physicians and specialists support better quality. Mechanisms that encourage doctors to think twice about prescribing invasive procedures promote better quality. Invasive procedures can put the patient at a higher risk than the original health condition did. A less costly, noninvasive treatment may be a better choice for the patient.

On the other hand, cost-control mechanisms that simply interfere with patients' getting the care they need clearly do not support higher quality. How can you, as a consumer who is not medically trained, know the difference? Stay tuned and we shall shed some light on this.

Like most myths, there's some truth to this one, but it is not entirely accurate.

Myth #3: "More Choice Equals Better Quality"

This myth reflects one of the most prevailing—yet inaccurate—beliefs about healthcare today. Most consumers assume that having more choices of physicians and hospitals in their

> Plans that allow unrestricted access to a broad selection of unrelated physicians, hospitals, and other providers do not have the infrastructure to promote the highest-quality care.

health plan is the best way to assure getting higher-quality care. The longer the list of available doctors and the fewer the restrictions on which doctors consumers can use, the higher the perceived quality of the health plan. After all, the plans with more choices tend to be more expensive, and we get what we pay for, don't we?

In truth, the health plans that support the highest-quality care are usually not composed of large networks of loosely coordinated physicians. Ironically, the more physicians and physician groups on a health plan's roster, and the fewer the restrictions on access to them, the more difficult it is for that health plan to ensure high-quality care. One major reason for this is that better care results from physicians practicing in well-integrated systems of care with good coordination and communication among primary-care and specialist physicians. Support services and ancillary providers are also part of these coordinated systems, and all physicians have access to fast-changing updates on proven treatment techniques.

Plans that allow unrestricted access to a broad selection of unrelated physicians, hospitals, and other providers do not have the infrastructure to promote the highest-quality care. Many health plans have extended their provider lists and dropped restrictions on direct access to a wide range of specialists solely to accommodate consumers' demands for greater freedom and choice. Therefore, consumer demand has, in part, led to a decrease in quality.

A few innovative health plans have taken a different approach. In certain parts of the country some health plans are providing information to their members comparing the quality of care of each of their participating medical groups and hospitals. As a result, many members switch to those medical groups and hospitals that rate highest in quality in the comparison reports.

The other medical groups and hospitals on the participating list have lost patients and are now paying more attention to improving the quality of care they provide in order to rate higher on the following year's report. Imagine if this happened everywhere in the country. Losing business is possibly the one thing that will give doctors and other providers the incentive to improve quality.

So, it isn't that *choice* is not good; it's just that having *greater numbers of choices* doesn't make your plan more valuable or improve the quality of care you'll receive. Choice is good. In fact, choice is essential to high-quality care. You have the freedom

> Losing business is possibly the one thing that will give doctors and other providers the incentive to improve quality.

and the right to choose healthcare providers who have demonstrated their competency. This is a much more meaningful way to think about choice than just to insist on longer lists.

With your new understanding, you can now choose healthcare plans and providers more effectively. You may even prefer plans with shorter lists if they offer providers who have demonstrated greater competency and higher-quality care. Furthermore, your insistence on having access to high-quality providers may, over time, encourage health plans to focus on offering access to only the better providers. This would decrease the plan's administrative costs as well as its costs of patient care, because the right care provided the first time saves overall costs. These cost savings could then be passed on to you.

These facts may come as a surprise to many consumers who, given the financial resources, pay more to participate in health plans with longer lists of easily accessible, unconnected physicians.

Keep an Open Mind

The myth that easy access to a broad selection of providers equals better quality is so pervasive that many of you may not believe me. Skepticism may keep you from obtaining the better-quality healthcare you really want. Let go of the preconceived notions you may be harboring—**PLEASE!**

Myth #4: "More Means Better"

Many people feel that, no matter what their symptoms or diagnosis, the quality of their care is in direct proportion to the amount of "stuff" they get. They think more is better. More office visits mean better care. If one test is needed, two tests are even better. If there is a more expensive drug available, it is probably the better one. And so on.

This is simply not so. Each patient's set of symptoms and risks warrants a proven care regimen—nothing more and nothing less. If one particular test or set of tests has been proven to be the best tool for diagnosing the suspected problem, that specific test or set of tests is the one you need—no more, no less. When drugs, unnecessary care, or invasive tests and surgeries can be avoided, they should be. Often, more "stuff" actually leads to greater illness, as when patients develop side effects from prescription drugs, get infections after being exposed to microbes in hospitals, or develop deep wound infections from invasive surgeries.

Myth-Understandings

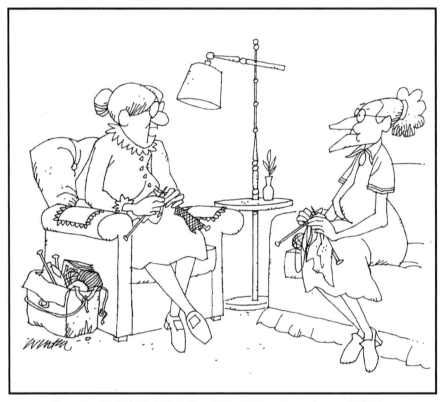

"AGNES, THIS AIDS BUSINESS MAKES ME THINK
WE SHOULD STOP SHARING NEEDLES."

If you are in the habit of thinking that more is better, no matter what the circumstances or symptoms, you have succumbed to a myth. Please change your thinking—you are not doing yourself any favors with this rationale. What you need is *scientifically proven* care, not simply more procedures, more drugs, extra tests, or more "stuff."

Myth #5: "Higher Cost Means Higher Quality"

The facts show that it is not correct to assume that doctors, hospitals, and other care providers who charge higher prices are giving better care than those who charge less. Some providers who charge less have proven that they give higher-quality care than some who charge the highest prices.

The connections between costs and quality care are complex. Some providers may charge more simply because they are perceived to be the premier providers in their market. However, general public perceptions about a provider's quality are not always justified. On the other hand, it does often require additional money to implement new high-quality care programs. The prices of those providers who are committed to high quality will include the costs of implementing these programs. But in the long run, better care often cuts a patient's overall costs by keeping the patient well and, when ill, by improving his or her health sooner with fewer complications.

So, unless you understand what to look for, you could pay top dollar and not get top value. The lesson: Learn what quality care looks like, use valid surveys to compare the quality of all providers available to you, and make choices based on true quality measures, not just cost.

Myth #6: "Doctor Welby Medicine Is Best"

A popular 1960s TV series featured Doctor Marcus Welby (played by actor Robert Young)—a wise, intelligent, kindly family physician in solo practice. Each heartwarming episode featured Dr. Welby taking good care of his patients. For many Americans, "Marcus Welby, MD" came to symbolize the best in American medical care. He epitomized our notions of what a family physician should be and do. Then and today, many of us wish he were our physician—someone we could trust to always take the very best care of us.

For those of you too young to remember the show, I'm sure you've seen plenty of movies where the trusted, kindly family doctor showed up at the house with his little black bag, ready to treat little Joseph or Sally for his or her malady.

We all want a doctor who has a kind, respectful, caring attitude. Wisdom in making decisions is also an attribute we should look for, and, of course, a physician must be highly intelligent to absorb the best medical knowledge and to use it well.

The problem with the myth "Doctor Welby Medicine Is Best" is that it promotes the solo practitioner as the symbol of the best in medical care. In addition, it promotes the myth that every physician who is kind and caring is providing high-quality medicine. To get the best in modern medicine, we need to recognize that excellent medical care now requires doctors to do many things they were not previously accustomed to doing.

Among other things, doctors need to keep pace with an astounding amount of new medical knowledge, as treatments quickly become outdated. In addition, doctors need to track large amounts of information about each patient accurately and routinely through sophisticated information systems. A physician practicing alone, outside of a strong support system, now has a much more difficult challenge in providing excellent medical care. Marcus Welby medicine may get us kindness, but it may not get us the highest-quality care.

> **A physician practicing alone, outside of a strong support system, now has a much more difficult challenge in providing excellent medical care.**

A physician's medical group can have a tremendous impact on that physician's ability to provide the best care. By banding together and pooling resources in medical groups, doctors can afford to hire extended professional support teams, including nutritionists, physical therapists, and nurse practitioners. Probably more importantly, large medical groups can afford to implement the costly electronic information and monitoring systems that support physicians in providing high-quality modern medicine (as explained fully in Part IV).

While it is possible for a physician practicing solo or in a less-supportive medical group to give high-quality care, it is much more difficult. My highest respect goes to those physicians who have mastered the quality challenges in spite of not having outside support. A number of these top-notch solo physicians practice in rural and semi-rural areas, where coming together with a larger number of physicians in a medical group is not possible. There are also some solo physicians practicing high-quality medicine even in urban areas where other physicians have banded together in larger groups to get better support.

Your challenge is to find a doctor who is committed to knowing and putting into practice the latest scientific guidelines, either through the assistance of electronic and other systems implemented by his or her medical group or through systems that are self-developed and self-administered.

Myth #7: "You Shouldn't Question What the Doctor Tells You"

One clear message that has come out of the best and most recent research on the quality of medical care in America is that *quality varies*—a lot—far more, in fact, than most of us realize. This means each of us must question the quality of care we are getting.

Traditionally, the doctor was the one who knew medicine and who was considered the "expert." Patients relied entirely on their doctor's advice and diagnosis. In fact, "advice" was prescriptive—like orders from on high—and went unchallenged. The doctor's word was gospel.

This myth lives on today, perpetuated by doctors who seem to resent being asked questions. Unfortunately, many feel they simply don't have time to deal with patients' questions or concerns about diagnoses, treatment options, or prescribed treatments. Overly compliant patients also perpetuate this myth. Some social researchers speculate that many patients want their physician to function as a "shaman," imbued with magical powers. However, patients need to take ownership of their health and well-being. After all, we, not our doctors, are most heavily vested in our bodies.

Even when the highest-quality care is being given, patients recover better when they really understand their health problems. Patients recover even better, in general, when they not only understand their medical condition but also understand all the options for treatment and participate in deciding on the best treatment.

It may seem easier for us to relinquish accountability and put all the responsibility for our well-being on our doctor. If he or she screws up, we can sue! Never mind that we may die younger or suffer some serious disability. But which would you rather have—good health or the right to blame someone else for poor health? Think about it.

Living in the Information Age, those of us who take responsibility for our health have a great deal of data available to us. Vast amounts of information, easily accessible via the Internet, can help us figure out what questions to ask about our diagnosis and find out about our medical care treatment options. With this information we are in a position to insist on partnering with our doctors to get our questions answered

> Always ask your doctor, "What preventive care or screenings should I be getting?"

and, when appropriate, to suggest or seek out treatment different from a doctor's recommendations.

Myth #8: "Your Doctor Will Tell You About All the Medical Care You Need to Stay Healthy"

Not only should you question any prescriptions or advice your doctor gives you, but you should also ask about information and prescriptions your doctor hasn't given you.

This is particularly true regarding preventive care. Research shows that consumers receive, on average, only 55% of the preventive care they should be getting.[2] This happens because physicians have many, many things to remember, and they tend to focus on whatever symptoms you have when you see them. Your doctor may simply forget to prescribe preventive care if she or he sees you only when you are ill. Always ask your doctor, "What preventive care or screenings should I be getting?" Better yet, ask your doctor to help you identify your disease risks and then investigate reliable sources, including those listed in Chapter 7, to find out for yourself. Then work with your doctor to make sure you get all the preventive care you need.

Recent research also confirms that many people who are being treated for chronic diseases, such as asthma and diabetes, are not receiving appropriate treatment.[3] If you have a chronic disease, find out what the recommended treatment is, based on the latest scientific evidence of what works best. Then work with your doctor to make sure you get that treatment. See Chapter 12 for more details.

The chart below summarizes the myths discussed in this chapter.

Eight Myths Dispelled

Myth	Truth
1. It's all the insurance companies' fault.	The whole system is in crisis, and everyone in the system shares responsibility for it, not just the insurance companies.
2. HMOs and other health plans impose controls on doctors and members solely to save money, with little regard for quality of care.	Some control mechanisms are purely for cost containment, but others promote higher quality. Some promote both quality and cost control at the same time.

Myth	Truth
3. Plans that offer more choices of physicians and hospitals are higher in quality.	A system that supports the highest-quality medical care is not composed of large networks of loosely coordinated providers. Quality results from physicians practicing in well-integrated systems with excellent coordination and communication among primary-care and specialist physicians and all other providers of care.
4. More care means better care.	Each patient's set of symptoms and risks warrants a proven care regimen—nothing more or less.
5. Higher cost means higher quality.	Higher cost and higher quality do not always go hand in hand. High quality sometimes means lower cost, and high cost does not guarantee high quality.
6. "Doctor Welby" medicine is best.	Modern medicine has advanced far beyond what was known in the 1960s. A physician practicing alone, outside of a strong support system, faces huge challenges in providing the best medical care. Many physicians practicing solo have not been able to keep up and may not be providing the best care. And kindness does not guarantee high-quality care.
7. The doctor's word is gospel.	The evidence shows that it is risky to relinquish responsibility for our own health. We must ask questions and seek information whenever necessary to make sure we and our doctors know the latest scientific evidence on the best treatment options. Then we need to work in partnership with our doctors to make decisions about treatment.

Myth	**Truth**
8. Your doctor will tell you about all the care you need.	Research shows that your doctor may not be telling you about the preventive care or the chronic disease management care you should be getting. Find out this information for yourself, then work with your doctor to be sure you get the care you need.

Jane

Sarah, a 30-year-old mother of one son, lives in a suburb of a very large city in the Midwest. Though she is in fairly good health herself, she worries about her mother's health. Jane, Sarah's mother, who lives in another nearby suburb, has diabetes. As a result of diabetes, Jane has already had some serious health problems and been hospitalized twice due to complications.

At a party recently, Sarah met Iris, whose father also has diabetes. His health had been failing badly for many years when he finally found a doctor who is part of a new program for doctors specializing in treating this disease. Since Iris's father started seeing this new physician, his health has improved dramatically. Unfortunately, Iris's father lives on the East Coast, so it would not be reasonable for Sarah's mother to see his doctor. However, Iris suggested that Sarah and her mother go to the National Committee for Quality Assurance website (*www.ncqa.org*) for a list of local doctors participating in the Diabetes Physician Recognition Program (listed under Recognized Physicians, Diabetes).

That evening when Sarah got home, she went to the website and found the names of two doctors in the program who practiced in the local metropolitan area. Sarah called her mother and suggested Jane see one of these two doctors to find out if he could help her better manage her diabetes. Jane resisted. She had been seeing her current doctor for about 20 years, and she liked him. She did not want to hurt his feelings by seeing another doctor. So, she thanked Sarah for the suggestion but said she would not change doctors.

Three weeks later, one of Jane's long-time friends died at age 62 after suffering and being disabled for years from complications of diabetes. Among other things, her friend had her right leg amputated just below the knee because of circulation problems, and she was on regular kidney dialysis treatment that severely restricted her activities. Lately, Jane had been feeling like her own condition was getting worse again and feared having the same complications of diabetes her friend had suffered. Jane adored her grandson, David, an energetic and charming three-year-old. She had enjoyed him as a toddler and wanted to be around to see him grow up. She thought about how her late friend would miss watching her own grandchildren grow. So, Jane reluctantly decided to make an appointment with one of the doctors Sarah had found.

At her first appointment, the doctor explained some things to Jane about her condition that she had never been told before. The doctor also matched Jane with a nurse to be her coach in keeping her condition under control. The nurse taught Jane how to better manage her diabetes at home. With good coordination between the doctor, the nurse coach, and Jane, over the next six months Jane began to feel better than she had in years. This was clearly the result of Jane's getting the help she needed to keep her blood sugar level under control.

5 All Doctors and Health Plans Are Not Created Equal

Learning without thought is labor lost. Thought without learning is perilous. —Confucius

In This Chapter...
- Typical, but problematic, ways many people choose their physicians.
- Why these methods don't necessarily lead to high-quality healthcare.
- Little specific information is available to consumers about the level of quality a physician provides.
- The types of physician-specific data that ARE available.

Most consumers don't understand how the healthcare system really works, and because of that, many choose their doctors in ways that don't yield the best results. For example, as you just read, Jane at first insists on staying with her original doctor even though he has not helped her control her diabetes as well as he could have. Not knowing what to look for, most consumers blindly trust their doctors to do the right thing. Unfortunately, valid studies show that the right thing often doesn't happen.

Wrong Reasons for Choosing Your Doctor

Right now, let's take a quick look at the ways in which many people choose their doctors. My goal is to point out how heavily most consumers rely on traditional methods that no longer make sense in the face of current evidence. I call these traditional ways "false starts," and millions of people use them.

1. The "What Do My Friends Do?" Method

"Dr. Smith is my golf buddy's doctor. If he's good enough for Larry, he's good enough for me."

Without a better method for choosing a good physician, many of us simply rely on the recommendations of friends. Unfor-

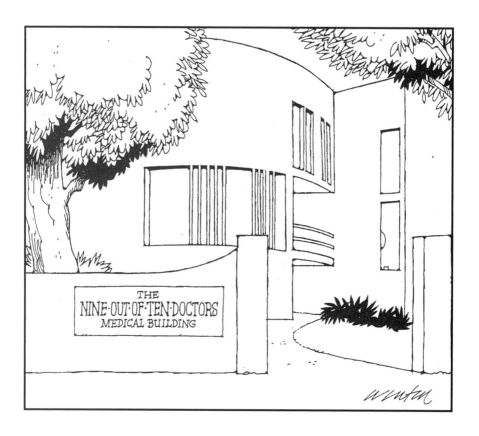

tunately, if our friends have not done their research, they may be making incorrect assumptions about the quality of care they are getting. By taking their advice, we end up making the same false assumptions.

2. The "Yellow Pages" Method

Man looking in phone book: *"Let's see here...which doctor should I choose? Adams, Abrahms, Ai, Bose, Brown, Crusoe, Diaz, Donley, Ellis.... I'll pick Dr. Ellis. His ad says he is one of the country's finest internists, and he's just down the block from my office!"*

Choosing a doctor from the phone book is as good a method as pulling a name out of a hat—no assurance of quality, even if the doctor's ad in the phone book says there is.

3. The "Frills" Method

"I look for expensive furniture and quality magazines in the waiting room. I figure if he can afford nice furniture, he must be a good doctor."

As you will see in the pages to come, neither cost of care nor waiting-room accessories are good measures of quality of care.

4. The "Nice Guy" Method

"He's really a nice guy. He reminds me of Dr. Welby."

A good "bedside manner" is a great attribute for a physician to have, but it does not guarantee quality of care.

5. The "He Gives Me Whatever I Want" Method

"Every time I ask for antibiotics, he gives me a prescription—no questions asked."

This is a complex but important issue. Giving you whatever you want, especially antibiotics too often or other care that can cause problems later, is not high-quality care. It is merely a way to avoid saying "No" to you or to avoid taking the time and effort to explain why what you are asking for is not good for you.

Overuse of antibiotics, for example, happens all too often and contributes to the development of bacteria that are resistant to the remedy. If you or your family members take antibiotics when you don't really need them, they may not be effective when you do need them. For example, many people assume that they should get antibiotics whenever they have a bad cold. But, in fact, antibiotics have no effect whatsoever on colds because colds are caused by viruses, and antibiotics have no impact on viruses.

Look for a doctor who practices in a setting that gives him or her the best available staffing, quality control, and information support systems.

One person I read about had gotten her doctor to prescribe antibiotics every time she had a cold. Then she developed a very serious infection from a paper cut that, as a result of her taking too many antibiotics previously, was resistant to almost every antibiotic that was tried as a cure. She went through weeks of disabling illness that could have been avoided if her doctor had had the courage to say "No" to her earlier requests. The federal Centers for Disease Control reports that 70% of the bacteria that cause hospital-acquired infections are now resistant to at least one antibiotic.[1]

So, you can see that you must be wise about what you demand from your doctor. And your doctor should be wise about what he or she agrees to give you.

The Ideal Physician

When seeking a new physician, look for a Dr. Welby—male or female—who is either part of a highly rated, highly integrated medical group, or who specializes in the type of treatment you need for a particular diagnosis (e.g., diabetes, heart disease, etc.). Make sure that he or she has proven competency in that specialty. Look for a doctor who practices in a setting that gives him or her the best available staffing, quality control, and information support systems. Relatively few physicians have all of these support systems available to them. Later chapters in this book will give you a better understanding of these systems so you will know what to look for.

What Does a Doc Want in a Doc?

Here is a list, given to me by a thoughtful, quality-minded physician, of the attributes she looks for when finding a physician for herself:

1. Keeps up with changing medical practice.

Scientific research continuously increases the medical knowledge base of what treatments work best for a given diagnosis. This knowledge base has grown exponentially over the last few decades and continues to expand at a mind-numbing pace, making it difficult for physicians to keep up. According to recent studies, only a minority of physicians actually incorporate the latest medical guidelines into their treatments for all diagnoses.

2. Makes wise decisions. Is moderately conservative in treatment—not the first to use new treatments and not the last.

Only about 30% of all the medical care provided by doctors has been clearly proven effective through scientific evidence. Some would say that estimate is too high. An even smaller percentage of treatment regimens have been subjected to randomized controlled scientific trials, which some medical experts say are required to actually prove the value of a treatment.

Even when physicians think they have "evidence," for example, when the FDA approves a drug for a particular medical condition, problems still crop up when the use is extended from a carefully controlled clinical trial to the real world. Some very high-profile drug recalls bring that point home. Therefore, many doctors believe that unless the situation is desperate—that is, unless there are no other options—it is best to wait until a drug has been out for a while before incorporating it widely into their practice. Of course, you don't want a physician who never gets around to using a new therapy or who is the last one to use it either.

3. Uses information technology to manage his or her practice. Has all needed information easily accessible to make a good decision.

Ideally, every physician should have access to a fully electronic set of medical records for every patient. This technology is not yet widely available. Short of that, there are a number of electronic systems that are readily available and extremely helpful. They provide:

· Electronic access to all diagnoses (including allergies), lab results, and prescriptions.

· Access to a patient-maintained electronic history.

4. Builds in consultation with respected colleagues—is not afraid to ask for help.

This doctor knows the limits of his or her expertise.

5. Knows about me—my life, my preferences, my work, etc. Works with me to make decisions about my care that fit my life.

6. Explains all of my conditions and the options for treatment—the upsides and downsides of each—and helps support me in making decisions that are right for me.

7. Is accountable to me and to society for high-quality, affordable care.

This means being willing to publicly report the cost and quality of care he or she provides so consumers can use this information in decision-making.

8. Is nice. (*Note that this is #8, not #1.*)

Available Data for Wisely Choosing a Physician[2]

The unfortunate truth is that there is not much physician-specific data available that can inform consumers about the level of quality a physician provides. We have few easy ways to find out whether a physician is up-to-date on the most effective therapies, or more importantly, if a physician actually applies this information, even if he or she knows it. Applying current medical information appropriately often requires using a database to track data about each patient.

To properly evaluate the level of quality a physician provides, we would need to know several important things:

1. What is the level of knowledge he or she has about the latest medical research?

2. Does he or she have access to good reminder systems for using this research?

3. Does he or she have access to—and does he or she use—good patient database systems?

In California, the Pacific Business Group on Health provides results to the public of a consumer survey rating the quality of care of 128 medical groups across the state. (See *www.healthscope.org.* Also available at *www.opa.ca.gov.*) Unfortunately, this type of information is not available in most other parts of the country. Even where information on the quality of medical groups is available, often that information does not compare the care of individual doctors. This is an important point, because even in high-performing medical groups, some doctors will be more diligent in quality practices than others.

"Best Doctors" lists are published annually by certain organizations. However, these lists usually only provide information about a doctor's training, location, and which hospitals and health plans he or she is affiliated with. Before relying on these types of lists, take the time to learn the basis of their rankings.

Five Good Ways to Find a Great Doctor

1. **Provider Recognition Programs**: The American Diabetes Association and the National Committee on Quality Assurance (NCQA) have a Provider Recognition Program that measures how well specific physicians and medical groups deliver high-quality diabetes care, based on the most up-to-date medical research. If you have, or a family member has, diabetes, contact one of the physicians on this list for care. You will find the list at *www.ncqa.org*. At that website, do a search for Diabetes Physician Recognition Program. The American Heart Association/American Stroke Association and NCQA are also developing a Heart/Stroke Recognition Program that will be designed in the same way to recognize physicians and medical groups delivering high-quality care for heart disease and stroke patients.

   Look for a physician who is Board Certified in the specialty area of your needs.

2. **Board Certification**: If a physician is Board Certified, it means that he or she has done additional training in and has passed tests on a medical specialty area. Tests are sponsored by an organization appropriate for that subject area, such as the American Academy of Pediatric Medicine. Therefore, physicians who are Board Certified are often better trained and more knowledgeable than those who are not. Look for a physician who is Board Certified in the specialty area of your needs. Many boards now require periodic recertification. Patients should ask if their doctor has recently been recertified in his or her specialty.

3. **Interaction With Patients**: The way a doctor interacts with patients is one key to the quality of care he or she gives. Doctors who communicate poorly or who don't take time to answer questions are not providing good patient care. Doctors who take the additional step of including the patient in decision-making are providing better care than those who don't.

   Patient feedback on how well a physician communicates, answers questions, and is willing to work in partnership with a patient is available from a few sources. Look for descriptions of individual physician "practice style and philosophy." You can always make an initial visit with

Finding a Good Doctor

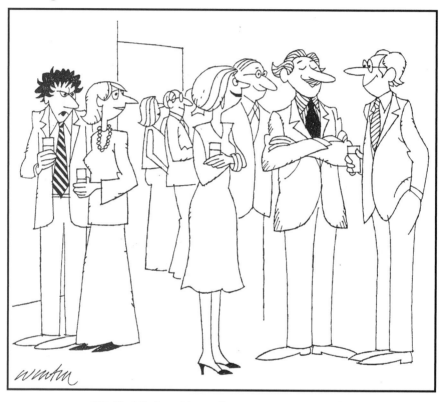

"IF HE'S SUCH A BRILLIANT DOCTOR,
WHY DOESN'T HE HAVE HIS OWN T.V. SHOW?"

a doctor to determine his or her style and then switch to another physician if that doctor doesn't meet your needs.

4. **Specialization in Specific Diagnoses or Treatments**: Some physicians choose to specialize in specific diagnoses or procedures, such as heart transplants. If you have a specific diagnosis and need treatment, you may receive better care from a doctor experienced in treating your diagnosis. However, it would still benefit you to research for yourself what the most up-to-date medical information shows to be the best treatment. To find guidelines for treatment of your diagnosis that are based on the latest scientific evidence, go to *www.guideline.gov*. Use this information to check whether your physician or intended physician knows and uses these guidelines.

5. **Participation in a Highly Rated Medical Group**: If medical groups in your geographic area have been researched and rated for quality by a trustworthy organization using criteria based on parameters such as those established by the National Committee on Quality Assurance, choose a physician from one of the highly rated groups. These groups choose their physicians carefully, and they monitor and provide support to participating physicians in order to keep the quality of care high.

Use caution if you find an organization that seems to provide quality comparison information on individual physicians. For example, one Internet site, *www.healthgrades.com*, lists 70% of all physicians as "leading physicians," largely based on the fact that these physicians have been Board Certified. Board Certification shows that a physician has increased his or her knowledge in a specific medical area. However, it does not prove that he or she knows and uses the latest research on the best medical practices.

See Appendix B for sources of lists of physicians.

Three Things to Consider in Selecting a Health Plan

Beyond being able to find a good doctor on a health plan's list, what factors are important in choosing one plan over another? Three questions are key to ask yourself:

1) Will I stay healthy better with one health plan versus another? In other words, how well will I get the preventive care that sound medical research has proven to be effective?

A number of factors go into answering this question.

- If you have a choice, the health plan you choose should cover all important preventive care at no or low out-of-pocket costs.

- The right plan for you will cover the particular preventive screening tests you need based on your risk factors. Only by knowing your risk factors and which tests you need will you be able to tell if a plan properly covers your preventive care. (See Chapter 7 for further details.)

- Next is whether you can find a doctor in the health plan who makes sure his or her patients get all appropriate preventive care.

- Some health plans assist their doctors in various ways to encourage them to give all needed preventive care. Some plans also send reminders to members, through newsletters or otherwise, to encourage using proven preventive screening tests. The National Committee for Quality Assurance (NCQA) website at *www.ncqa.org* has comparative information on how well health plans are preventing certain major diseases.

2) When I am sick, will I get the best care possible?
   Consider the following factors to answer this question.
   - Choosing your primary-care and specialist physicians is key here. You must read the rest of this book to see why. Many issues are involved, and not necessarily the ones you think.

   - Choosing a health plan should be based on how well the health plan gives you access to physicians, hospitals, and other providers who rate highly in valid quality comparison surveys. Beware of general public perceptions about the quality of a specific health plan, hospital, or any other provider. These perceptions can be wrong. Read the rest of this book and check out the resources listed in Appendix B for more information on this.

   - Some health plans do better than others in helping their doctors coordinate the care of chronically and seriously ill patients. Some case management and disease management programs are better than others. See Chapter 12 for details. And see the National Committee for Quality Assurance (NCQA) website at *www.ncqa.org*. It has comparative information on not only how well health plans are preventing certain major diseases but also how well their doctors treat certain diseases.

- Your total costs for any care you may need are also important. You must understand and compare what your care will cost in each of your health plan options. Balance the projected costs against the level of quality you will receive. You must read the rest of this book to know the details of how to judge quality and cost-effectiveness in healthcare choices.

3) When I need medical care, either preventive care to stay well or care when I am sick, will I be able to get that care easily? The following access-to-care factors should be considered in comparing health plans. If care is not convenient, you may be tempted to avoid getting needed care.

- Is the location of the providers convenient for you, including laboratory and pharmacy?

- Are the office hours of the providers and the health plan member assistance services convenient?

- How easily can you get through by phone to your key providers and health plan member assistance?

- If you and/or covered family members need to speak to physicians and other providers in a language other than English, how well does your health plan and the providers it offers accommodate your language needs?

Consider Your Approach

Using the resources in Appendix B, seek out existing unbiased studies that make quality comparisons among medical groups, hospitals, and health plans in your area. *If you find that there aren't any studies for your area, take the time to let your physician and health plan know that you want them to begin participating in such research.*

Then, you must act—speak to the people to whom you are considering entrusting your healthcare. In other words, interview them! Interview the top providers from the studies. Or use the quality-of-care signposts in Part IV to ask about your providers' commitment and ability to give you the highest-quality care. This means you may have to be more of an activist than you have been up to now.

Sadly, many physicians, hospitals, and other providers lack incentive to give the best care. Your insistence on improved quality can motivate them to raise the caliber of the care they provide. Though government regulations demanding compliance with quality standards might help, competition for customers who demand excellence will most certainly spur providers to continuously improve and seek innovations in quality.

Resources in this book that can help you: Part IV helps you understand the elements that define medical quality. In Part VI, Chapter 23 gives you a basic understanding of how cost relates to quality. Appendix A gives you resources for trustworthy information on medical conditions and treatments. Appendix B shows you how to obtain information comparing the quality of physicians, hospitals, and health plans in your area if such information is available.

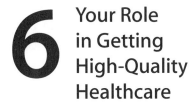

6 Your Role in Getting High-Quality Healthcare

Life shrinks or expands in proportion to one's courage.
—Anais Nin

In This Chapter...
- Research shows better outcomes of care when the patient is a full partner in the process.
- What it means to be a partner with your doctor.
- Suggestions for how to become a full participant on your healthcare team.

Now that we've dispelled some myths, answered some questions, and examined some common mistakes, you know how NOT to proceed. Without all that baggage holding you back or adding unnecessary confusion, you can proceed with a bit more forethought...and with a road map to guide you.

For Best Results, Get Involved in Your Care

According to the Institute of Medicine,[1] evidence shows that patients who understand their medical problems and who take responsibility for their treatment decisions experience better results than patients who leave such decisions to their doctors. Though not widely known, this is a major factor in maintaining the best health. The following are specific results for patients who participate in making decisions about their healthcare:

• Their medical conditions show more improvement.

• The total cost of their care is less.

• Their overall ability to function normally is greater.

Institute of Medicine Favors Patients As Decision-Makers

Twenty-one studies published between 1983 and 1993 measured how doctor–patient communication affected patient health for conditions such as breast cancer, diabetes, peptic ulcer disease, hypertension, and headaches.[2] High-quality doctor–patient communication was defined as leading to better-informed patients who actively participated in decisions about their healthcare. The results?

- 16 studies reported better health results for patients with high-quality doctor–patient communication than for those with poorer doctor–patient communication

- 4 studies reported positive (but not significant) results

- 1 study was inconclusive

Due to this and other evidence, the Institute of Medicine recommends that: *"Except in unusual circumstances, control should reside with patients."*

> A good doctor will respect your determination to be well informed so that you can actively participate in the decision-making process.

Be Proactive

Think about how our healthcare system would change if the role of the consumer shifted from "passive subordinate" to "researcher/decision-participant." How can we make this happen? In an ideal world, our doctors would spend all the time and effort necessary to educate us about each diagnosis, its causes, treatment options, side effects, and so forth. In today's world, the reality is that most doctors just can't take time to do this. However, a doctor could point us to easily accessible sources of complete and accurate information. Simply ask your doctor where you can find the information you need. If your doctor doesn't offer any help, research your diagnosis and science-based recommended treatments by using the Appendices in this book or other reliable sources.

Where to Get More Information

Even if you get information from your physician, you need to make sure the information is complete. A good doctor will respect your determination to be well informed so that you can actively participate in the decision-making process. One doctor I know says he never has enough time in office visits to give his patients all the information they should have about their diseases, yet he fully believes, based on his experience, that patients who have a greater understanding of their conditions do better. This doctor is pleased when his patients research their diseases on their own, using trustworthy sources, and then come to him with questions they have after doing the research.

As many of you already know, a vast amount of information is now available on the Internet and in other publicly accessible databases. In fact, thousands of Americans are already using the Internet to gather medical information. The biggest challenge with using the Internet this way is in knowing which websites to trust. Appendix A lists trustworthy websites that were current at the time this book went to press.

To determine the credibility of a site, you need to look for bias. For example, a key thing to watch out for is whether the site ultimately wants to sell you something—such as a site that is sponsored by a drug company. Beware—sometimes the site's commercial nature is carefully hidden. Generally, government sites are the most trustworthy and comprehensive, though those of some respected medical organizations (such as the Mayo Clinic and others) are also excellent. If you use trustworthy sites, there is a tremendous amount of useful information on the Net.

Your local library can also be a good source of information. A librarian can help you locate the information you need. In addition, there are three kinds of special medical libraries you can check:

- **Medical school libraries:** Some medical schools allow the public to use their libraries. Though you can't always check material out, you may be able to find data on specific topics.

- **Health plan libraries:** Some health plans maintain libraries of medical journals and other trustworthy data sources.

- **Medical data libraries:** In some large cities, special medical data libraries exist to assist the public in getting good and complete information about medical diagnoses and treatments, and sometimes even about alternative medical care that is outside the established medical care system.

They're YOUR Records

In the past, patients were not allowed to see their medical records. Physicians guarded patient files in an effort to maintain control. They assumed that patients would be unduly frightened or would misunderstand the information.

Demand Respect and Partnering

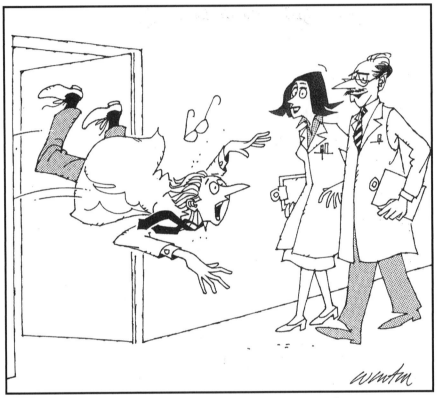

"LOOKS LIKE PETER'S HAVING A LITTLE TROUBLE
WITH PATIENT SATISFACTION AGAIN."

Now, by law, patients can see their medical records *upon request*. However, many consumers don't even think about asking. Tell your doctor you'd like to see your file. Go through it and make sure you understand everything in it and ask questions about anything you do not understand. When you have any tests done, ask for a copy of the results report.

In addition to knowing what is in your medical records, you need to keep track of your medical history. Keep records of your health events, family history of illnesses, dates of immunizations, and copies of lab reports. Make lists of current and past medications with dosage levels and frequencies, and note any side effects or allergies you have experienced due to specific treatments or drugs. Give a copy of your records to a family member or trusted friend to give to a new healthcare provider in the case of a medical emergency. You can also give a copy of your personal records to any new doctor treating you—as a way to make efficient use of your time together as well as to start the partnership off right.

> Now, by law, patients can see their medical records *upon request.*

Stand Up For Yourself

Whenever a person takes full responsibility for his or her health, learning about the diagnosis and researching treatment options, there is always the possibility that he or she may choose to vary from recommended treatment. This becomes a problem when scientific evidence clearly shows one treatment to be the best. Nonetheless, the patient may feel strongly about trying a different treatment. In our current system, as long as the patient pays any extra costs, this is allowed, as it should be.

Here's an example. If a patient elects to have a procedure that hasn't yet been proven (an "experimental" procedure, let's say) and that is not covered by his or her plan—he or she usually must pay all costs of the procedure. This can be very expensive for the patient or the patient's family, but may seem to be the only good alternative in some situations. Additionally, if this is the route you choose, you may have to find a doctor outside of your health plan to give you the treatment.

But what if the treatment you have chosen has been proven to be more effective, or equally effective but less risky, than the one your health plan is willing to pay for? Then being outraged at the health plan is justified, and you should protest the plan's decision. Most states now have laws protecting consumers in this situation. Some states have special agencies that help consumers resolve problems with their health plans. Check with your state government if you need this type of assistance.

Special Situations

In some situations patients are unable to make good decisions for themselves. Thus, the extent to which patients participate in their care must be based on each individual's circumstances. Here are two examples where someone other than the patient needs to partner with the doctor in making decisions:

> Remember, your relationship with your doctor should be a partnership!

- **Mental incapacity:** A patient may not be able to think clearly about his or her health situation. This could be a result of actual mental incapacity or of such intense pain as to render the person incapable of making a rational decision at the time.

- **Children:** Parents must obviously make decisions for very young children. As children get older, though, parents can begin to develop responsibility in their children by involving them in the decisions about their healthcare. The benefits of this are worth any challenges it creates.

Except in these special situations, all patients should participate in making decisions about their own care. Today, the norm in the majority of U.S. medical establishments is for the doctor to be the sole decision-maker about a patient's care. However, because the evidence shows that better health results when patients are partners in the decision-making process, this attitude must be challenged. Many patients are inexperienced in the role of decision-maker and will need coaching and encouragement. Even for those who resist investing time to research and ponder every medical decision, being a partner in decision-making is crucial when a serious illness is involved.

Prepare for When You Can't Make Decisions

When patients are unable to participate in making decisions about their care, giving such authority to a family member or trusted friend is often a better alternative to handing over all power to the doctor. To prepare for this, each of us should have an Advance Directive legal document. *Advance Directive* is a term that applies to legal documents of two types. These documents may be called by different names, such as a Living Will or Medical Power of Attorney. All such documents allow you to give instructions about how you want to be cared for and/or who should make decisions for you if you are unable to do so yourself because of illness or disability.

You can find good information about these legal documents as well as state-specific, blank Advance Directive documents at the website of the non-profit organization Partnership for Caring (*www.partnershipforcaring.org*). You can download the documents and their instructions free from the website, or you can call 1-800-989-9455 to order state-specific documents for $10 plus applicable tax, paying by credit card. The documents themselves as well as the directions for completing them vary from state to state.

I encourage you, for the sake of your health, to get the information you need and to insist on working with your doctor to make decisions about your healthcare—no matter what it takes. Ask the necessary questions and seek the necessary data to truly understand the issues and your options for treatment.

Some patients have the added challenge of a language barrier. Others find it difficult to understand complex medical information. Under these circumstances you may need to ask even more questions until you understand exactly what the information means. Some feel uncomfortable questioning their doctors, especially when the doctor is reluctant to spend time or to share information. Some of us do not feel comfortable challenging our doctor when he or she insists on making the decisions for us. For the best health results, we need to overcome all of these barriers.

How to Talk With Your Doctor[3]

Talking with your doctor can be challenging. Many of us feel rushed and sometimes intimidated by our doctors. We often walk away from a doctor visit feeling vulnerable and confused and with questions still unanswered. Communicating well is critical to getting good care. Remember, your relationship with your doctor should be a partnership! The following tips can help you be assertive and take an active role in improving your healthcare.

Remember Who You Are

Remember that you are the client and your doctor is your paid medical consultant. You are paying for his or her time and expertise. Don't allow your doctor to rush or interrupt you. Don't be either passive or aggressive. Be assertive.

Give Information; Don't Wait to Be Asked

To get the best from your doctor and your visit, bring an up-to-date "health history" list with you. Include significant medical care you have received as well as your current symptoms, stated very specifically. Bring two copies, as your doctor will probably want one for your file.

Always be completely honest with your doctor about your needs and concerns and about any aspects of your life that could be important—even if you feel embarrassed or uncomfortable.

You cannot just blindly accept advice from any physician.

Keep a journal of events related to your health problem. For example, if you have high blood pressure, take your blood pressure at home regularly and, in your journal, keep track of the readings. Always write down any unusual symptoms in your journal. Be as specific as possible. For example, instead of writing "I feel feverish today," write "Today my temperature was 101 degrees." Instead of writing "I'm very thirsty," write "I drank 4 liters of water today, and I'm still thirsty." Bring a printout or copy of the relevant pages of your journal each time you visit your doctor. Ask him or her to put the pages in your medical chart.

To every doctor visit, always bring any medicines you are taking, or at least a list of them, with data on the dosages and frequency of use. Include all over-the-counter, herbal, and alternative medicines you take either regularly or occasionally, as any of these could interact negatively with a medication your doctor may prescribe.

Tell your doctor about any alternative treatments you receive.

Bring other medical information, such as x-ray films, test results, and medical records.

If you have a serious illness and have researched your condition, bring printouts of any published material you have that you want your doctor to consider or discuss with you. For best results, do not take this material with you to your appointment. Instead, fax/mail/deliver the material beforehand with a cover note saying that you'd "like to discuss this at our next appointment, on (date)." Make sure you read the material thoroughly yourself. You will more likely get your doctor's respect and attention if you have looked up all unfamiliar terms in advance and if you are able to intelligently discuss the key points of the articles.

Get Information

Ask questions until you thoroughly understand your medical problem, everything your doctor says about it, and everything about the medications and treatments he or she is prescribing.

If you have questions before the visit, write them down. List the most important ones first. Fax or mail them to your doctor ahead of the visit if your time with your doctor tends to be rushed. Tell your doctor at the beginning of the visit that you have questions so that she or he will be sure to leave time for them.

Take notes on what your doctor says during the visit. Some people find it easier to remember information if they tape-record the visit and listen to the tape later. But always ask if it's OK to tape-record. If you need to, ask your doctor to draw pictures to help explain something.

You might want to bring someone along to help you ask questions. This person can also help you understand and/ or remember the answers.

Let your doctor know if you need more time to ask questions. If your doctor does not have time to extend your visit, ask to speak to a nurse or physician assistant. Or ask if you can call later to speak with someone.

A Minimum of Effort Can Make a Maximum of Difference

My life, like yours, is very busy. Unless I become extremely ill, I don't want to have to spend hours researching every little health concern I have. For people like me, the answer is to use reliable sources of data to find a trustworthy, high-quality physician. Once you find that doctor, work with him or her to make sure you get all your questions answered. Make sure you feel comfortable about your relationship and his or her commitment to providing high-quality care—then trust him or her to give you the best advice and treatment for promoting your health. However, you must have solid reasons to trust a physician. You cannot just blindly accept advice from any physician. Taking responsibility for your health entails **at least doing the following**:

- Know your health risk factors and what preventive care you need, and make sure you get all recommended preventive care. (See Chapter 7.)

- Have at least a basic understanding of your medical conditions, your treatment options, and why a particular treatment option is recommended.

- Know and follow through on the behaviors (e.g., exercise, diet, etc.) that will support your best health. (See Chapter 8.)

Some Pitfalls

I wrote this book to encourage you to proactively take ownership of your health and healthcare. However, I want to pass on some caveats. It is possible to take this notion too far and put yourself at increased risk. Keep the following in mind as you become more actively involved in your healthcare.

- **PLEASE do *not* self-diagnose or determine the treatments you need.** Some consumers use information from the Internet and other sources to self-diagnose and determine the treatment they need. They then try to find a physician who will give them what they have decided they need. As ill-advised as taking on your own legal defense without a law degree, self-diagnosis and making treatment decisions on your own, without the years of training physicians receive, is extremely risky. It also makes it very difficult for your doctor to work with you effectively. Consumers who try to completely take over the doctor's legitimate role put themselves at increased risk. Rather, taking greater responsibility for partnering with your doctor will give you the greatest health results. This book will give you guidance to accomplish this goal.

- **Not all online information is reliable.** Though the Internet offers an incredible amount of medical information to the public, a significant part of this information is only partially valid or is inaccurate. The Appendix section lists reliable Internet sources of information.

- **Beware of non-approved online pharmaceuticals.** Purchasing drugs on the Internet from sources that may not be approved by the FDA is also dangerous. You can't really be sure what is in these drugs. They may not even contain active ingredients!

- **Don't make assumptions about the safety of combining prescribed or over-the-counter drugs with "natural" substances.** Taking natural remedies, such as "health-enhancing" herbs and supplements purchased from health food stores, in combination with prescribed or over-the-counter medications can cause negative interactions. Be sure to talk over the use of these products with your doctor or trusted pharmacist. Even combining over-the-counter drugs with prescribed drugs can be risky.

- **Be careful with the alternatives.** Experimenting with unproven alternative medicine therapies may produce negative side effects. Always consult your doctor before trying any new treatment.

Please be bold, but also wise, about taking responsibility for your health and healthcare.

Part III

Preventing a Problem Is Better Than Trying to Fix One

Chapter 7
Preventive Care: Avoiding Illness and Enhancing Quality of Life

Chapter 8
More Benefits of Prevention

Of all the sections in this book, Part III gives you the most important information about how to maximize your health. This information is most useful to those of you who are currently healthy. It also shows those of you who are ill how to avoid other kinds of illnesses and disabilities.

To get the best understanding of prevention, you need to know what the healthcare system should be providing you as well as what you should be doing for yourself.

Chapter 7 gives you a good overview of the preventive care and screening the healthcare system should give you. Too often, even well-insured individuals do not get the screening tests they should be getting. Find out what you need and be sure you get it.

Chapter 8 gives you information that will have more impact than anything else in this book on how long you live, how ill you will be, and how disabled you will be in your later years. Whether you are currently well or ill, please read this chapter and take it seriously.

Joe

Five years ago, Susan married Joe. Joe, 45, is a big guy—6 feet tall and 200 pounds. He's typical of many men in that he does not like to go to doctors and, in fact, had not seen a doctor in many years.

Recently, while waiting for an appointment in her dentist's office, Susan happened to read an article about men's health that listed the preventive care men should have at different ages and pointed out the medical problems that could result if preventive care was not received. This brought up Susan's long-standing worries about Joe's health. That night, Susan and Joe had a huge argument about Joe's ignoring his potential health problems. In fact, the argument went on for several days and threatened to cause a rift in their relationship. Joe finally reluctantly decided to go for a checkup. He got a doctor's name from his best friend since he did not know any doctors himself.

Though happy that Joe had an appointment, Susan was afraid that Joe would not be thorough in discussing his health with the doctor. She decided to make the most of his checkup by preparing a list of the preventive care he should ask the doctor about. The article she'd read had said to pay attention to personal risk factors, including family medical history, among other things, to determine what preventive care each person might need.

Joe's father had died about 15 years ago of colon cancer at age 63. The article said that colon cancer was easily cured if caught in its early stages, but that many people did not get the preventive screening in time. Sadly, many people die prematurely unnecessarily. Susan put a star beside "colon cancer screening" on the list she was preparing for Joe's checkup.

That made Susan think to ask Joe about other health problems his family might have had. She knew that Joe's mother, Isabell, suffered from heart problems, but did not know any of the details. She asked Joe about his mother's and other relatives' health problems. Joe said his father's brother had died from skin cancer, and several relatives suffered from arthritis. Susan even called Joe's mother, explained her project, and got further details about the family health history.

At his appointment, Joe sheepishly handed the doctor the clearly laid out list of preventive care he might need and the family history Susan had put together. Though Joe had been given a health history questionnaire to fill out when he got to the doctor's office, he did not have time to complete it before the nurse called him back to see the doctor. The doctor looked at Susan's list very carefully and said he was extremely impressed. He said Susan had made it possible for him to do a better job for Joe than he could normally do for most of his patients, since his schedule was often rushed and he had time to focus only on key health problems at each visit.

The doctor quickly wrote orders for lab tests as well as referrals to certain specialists for Joe to see. He explained that at Joe's age it was important to stay on top of potential health problems and that being thorough about preventive care was the right thing to do. The doctor remarked what a caring wife Susan had been to put together the list for Joe's checkup. Joe was pleased and decided to go straight to the lab for his tests. At first he thought about skipping the tests and doing them another day, but knew that if he didn't do them right then, he might put them off indefinitely.

Joe then went home and, chagrined, told Susan everything the doctor had said. He told her about the referrals to specialists, including one to a dermatologist to check two suspicious moles on his back. Susan scheduled Joe's appointment with the dermatologist for the next week. At his appointment, the dermatologist told Joe that both of the moles needed to be removed, and she performed the biopsy during the office visit. Two days later, she called Joe with the lab results: Joe had a developing malignancy in one mole, and a larger section needed to be taken out.

When Joe went back to have the larger section removed, the doctor told him that he was very lucky the problem had been caught before the malignancy became serious. She checked the rest of Joe's body for other skin problems, found none, but warned Joe that he was at high risk for more skin cancer and should be checked annually. She also asked Joe to encourage other family members to be checked, as this type of problem runs in families. Joe, shocked about the pre-malignancy, felt a huge wave of gratitude for Susan's thorough focus on illness prevention. He remembered how his uncle had suffered and had died too young from skin cancer. Joe did not want that to happen to him.

At Joe's follow-up visit with his primary-care doctor, the doctor suggested that Joe (or Susan) keep a running health history—keeping track of all of his test results and lab work, all medications, and all other health-related events. He said that everyone should do this—though few people do—not only for himself or herself, but also to share with every new doctor who treats him or her.

7 Preventive Care: Avoiding Illness and Enhancing Quality of Life

It's not the years in your life that count. It's the life in your years.
—Abraham Lincoln

I don't want to get to the end of my life and find that I have just lived the length of it. I want to have lived the width of it as well.
—Diane Ackerman

In This Chapter...
- Prevention is more important than many people realize.
- Preventing disability as we age is at least as important as preventing early death.
- Many people don't get the preventive care they should have.
- How you can be sure to get the preventive care you need.

Here is a staggering statistic: As many as 50% of all untimely deaths from chronic disease could be avoided through better preventive care. At least as important is the fact that much of the disease-related disability Americans now suffer could have been prevented, reduced, or delayed.[1] People are becoming disabled unnecessarily! Some of my older relatives are now suffering serious disabilities that could have been avoided through better preventive care. This really makes me angry and has been a major motivation in my writing this book.

Joe's story on the preceding pages shows how good preventive care can catch big problems early, preventing the onset of disease. In cases where there is no cure for the illness or it is not prevented entirely, such as if you have already developed heart disease, good management by your doctor can help you keep the disease under control so that it does not cause more major damage to your body.

High-quality healthcare providers, health systems, and health plans emphasize prevention and early treatment. This includes screening tests and education on healthful lifestyles and self-care. *This also includes careful monitoring of your condition even when you are being treated for a chronic disease, to make sure your treatment is working.* The preventive care approach results in better health for the consumer as well as lower expense overall. Not employing this approach is not only stupid, it is almost criminal in light of the costs in human suffering, dollars, and productivity that are incurred when these preventive measures are not provided.

Silent Killers

As many as 50% of all untimely deaths from chronic disease could be avoided through better preventive care.

Remember the story of Flora in Chapter 1? Many of us don't fully "get" the connection between the lack of prevention and the suffering of disabilities and/or early death down the road. This is apparent by the number of people who don't make sure they get preventive care. In some cases, like Flora's, we are essentially betrayed by our doctors, whom we trust to prescribe all the clinical preventive care we need. In far more cases, however, we know we need to quit smoking, lose weight, exercise more, etc., to decrease our risks of developing illness later in life. And we know there are probably prevention screening exams we need, but we put them off. But how many of us are truly aware of the risks we are taking? For example, how many of us realize the following?

- High blood pressure (hypertension) is a condition that has no symptoms. It puts stress on blood vessels, forcing the heart to overwork. High blood pressure hugely increases the risk of stroke, heart failure, and kidney disease. Heart disease, usually caused or aggravated by high blood pressure, is one of the leading preventable causes of death in the U.S.

- One in every five adults has high blood pressure (an estimated 50 million Americans).[2]

- Almost as many (about 45 million Americans) are "prehypertensive," having blood pressure levels that indicate they are at high risk for developing hypertension. New studies show that even at prehypertensive levels there is damage to arteries.[3]

- The vast majority of us will develop hypertension (high blood pressure). According to a study reported recently in the *Journal of the American Medical Association*, a 55-year-old with normal blood pressure today has a 90% lifetime chance of developing high blood pressure. High blood pressure is the most commonly diagnosed and treated condition in the U.S.[4]

- Yet 30% of people who already have hypertension do not know it. This is because it does not have any obvious symptoms and they have not had their blood pressure checked.[5]

- Only one of every three people with high blood pressure succeeds in lowering it to safe levels. This is partly because many people who have high blood pressure either don't follow through on the diet and exercise advice of their doctors or they don't take the prescribed medication regularly or they do not know they have a problem.[6] Unfortunately, this is also partly because some doctors who have patients with hypertension do not work diligently at getting their patients' blood pressure to target levels.[7]

- Effective treatment for hypertension reduces the risk of stroke by 35-40%, reduces the risk of heart attacks by 20-25%, and reduces the risk of congestive heart failure by 50%![8]

> **High-quality healthcare providers, health systems, and health plans emphasize prevention and early treatment.**

High blood pressure has been called the silent killer, but there are other diseases and conditions that have no symptoms in their early stages that can also be considered silent killers. High blood cholesterol, diabetes, and glaucoma are good examples. Most silent killer conditions can be detected through the appropriate clinical preventive screening and can be treated early. Many can be prevented altogether through healthy living.

You Can Beat the Odds

According to the Centers for Disease Control (CDC), the average life expectancy in the U.S. is over 75 years. A word to the wise: If you want to live and live well to at least 75 years of age, pay close attention to the paragraphs that follow.

The leading cause of death in the U.S. for people under 65 is cancer, according to the National Center for Health Statistics. Scientifically proven screening tests are available to detect various types of cancer in their early stages, when treatment is more effective. Some screening tests, such as colorectal cancer screening, actually detect and allow for removal of pre-cancerous lesions. Get the cancer screening tests and exams you should have. Look for information about these in this chapter, through your local library, or on the Internet sites listed in Appendix A. The screening tests and exams include cervical cancer checks (Pap smears), mammograms to detect breast cancer, skin cancer checks, and screening tests for colon cancer, among others.

The second leading cause of death for people under 65 is heart disease, and heart disease is the number one cause

The Advantages of Healthy Living

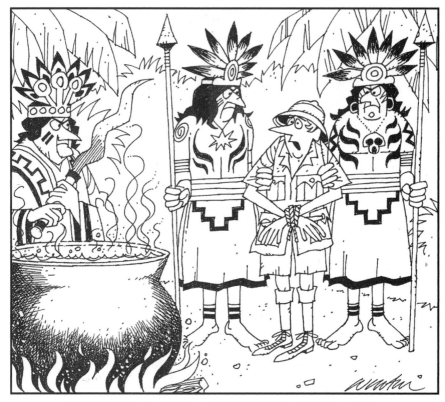

"BUT REALLY I WOULDN'T TASTE THAT GOOD.
MY CHOLESTEROL IS JUST 170."

of death for people over 65. See the discussion above about high blood pressure and look for more information on heart disease prevention below and on the Internet sites listed in Appendix A.

Those who contract cancer, heart disease, or other killer diseases but manage to survive to at least 65 may beat the survival statistics, but their quality of life is usually greatly impaired. The real trick is not just to survive the chronic disease killers but to avoid the diseases in the first place, or at least to catch them at very early stages.

> **Make sure you get the preventive care you need, so that you don't become unnecessarily disabled or die prematurely.**

Prevention Basics

The U.S. Preventive Services Task Force (USPSTF), sponsored by the Agency for Healthcare Research and Quality (AHRQ), is an independent panel of experts that reviews the evidence and develops recommendations for clinical primary-care and prevention services. The task force first issued recommendations for preventive care in its *Guide to Clinical Preventive Services*, first edition, in 1984. Those recommendations were updated in a second edition, published in 1996. The updates were based on research done after 1984 that showed where the old recommendations needed to be revised. A third edition is now in progress. Updates based on new recommendations are being released as they become available.[9]

All of this information, including the updates and a great deal of background data, is available to the public at the AHRQ website, *www.preventiveservices.ahrq.gov*, or by contacting AHRQ Publications Clearinghouse at:

P.O. Box 8547
Silver Springs, MD 20907
800-358-9295
410-381-3150 (callers outside the United States only)
888-586-6340 (toll-free TDD service, hearing impaired only)
Email: *ahrqpubs@ahrq.gov*

For a printed copy of the *Guide to Clinical Preventive Services*, second edition, ask for Publication OM97-0001. The price of a single copy as this book goes to press is $20. The publication number for the periodic updates is APPIP02-0001. The price of a subscription to the entire series of new task force recommendations and chapters is currently $60. However, you can print as much as the average person needs directly from the website for free.

To directly access a list of recommendations from the second edition of the *Guide to Clinical Preventive Services,* go to *www.ahrq.gov/clinic/cpsix.htm.* To directly access a list of the new recommendations from the third edition of the guide, go to *www.ahrq.gov/clinic/cps3dix.htm.* These recommendations are also released incrementally in a loose-leaf notebook available by subscription.

Most silent killer conditions can be detected through the appropriate clinical preventive screening and can be treated early. Many can be prevented altogether through healthy living.

Know Your Risks—Knowledge Is Power

Identifying our risk factors, which are based on age, sex, family history, lifestyle, etc., is key to preventing or curbing the onset of disease for each of us. In the current healthcare system, many of us turn over this responsibility to our doctors. A better, more "take charge" approach would be to talk with our doctors to get a clear understanding of all of our risk factors. For example, if your father and/or your mother has/had heart disease, then you need to find out about your risks for heart disease and how you can minimize them. Knowing and addressing your risks with a healthful lifestyle and appropriate preventive screening starting at age 30 will put you less at risk than if you wait to address your risks until age 50 or 60.

Go to *www.preventiveservices.ahrq.gov* for a complete list of the preventive services for your age group. Pay particular attention to preventive care for those health problems for which you are at highest risk.

You can also go to the websites of national organizations that focus on specific diseases, such as the American Heart Association, for assistance with your assessment and to get advice related to your risk. See Appendix A for names and websites of organizations that might be helpful. Some health plans may also provide risk assessment tools. Check your health plan's website to see what may be available to you.

A Summary of Recommended Preventive Services

The following table lists preventive screening tests, immunizations, preventive medications, and counseling interventions currently recommended by the U.S. Preventive Services Task Force.[10] Remember that these recommendations change over time, based on new research results. Be sure to check the AHRQ website for updates.

HEALTHCARE SERVICE	FOR	COMMENTS
Preventive Care: Immunizations		
Childhood Vaccines: • Oral poliovirus • Diphtheria-Tetanus-Pertussis • Measles-Mumps-Rubella • Haemophilus influenza type b • Hepatitis B • Varicella *See USPSTF website at www.preventiveservices.ahrq.gov for more detailed recommendations and age schedules for vaccinations.*	Children, by 18 months old and then at older ages as specified in USPSTF guidelines*	Largely as a result of widespread childhood vaccination over the past several decades, diphtheria, pertussis, tetanus, poliomyelitis, measles, mumps, rubella, and congenital rubella syndrome have become much less common in the U.S. The numbers of cases reported are at or near the lowest levels ever. Not receiving the immunizations puts children at risk of contracting potentially disabling diseases that are easily preventable.
Influenza Vaccine: Annual vaccination —*U.S. Preventive Services Task Force (USPSTF), 1989. Recommendation reiterated in 1996.* No changes to date.	All people 65+	Twenty thousand or more excess deaths have been reported during each of 10 different flu epidemics from 1972 to 1991. More than 40,000 excess deaths occurred in each of three of these epidemics. More than 90% of the deaths attributed to pneumonia and influenza in these epidemics occurred among persons aged 65+.
Pneumococcal (Pneumonia)Vaccine: Once only for all immunocompetent individuals. —*U.S. Preventive Services Task Force (USPSTF), 1996.* No changes to date.	All people 65+	Periodic revaccination may be appropriate for those with severe chronic disease who were vaccinated more than five years previously.
Cancer Screening		
Breast Cancer Screening: Screening mammography every one to two years, with	All women 40+	Breast cancer is the most common cancer among women in the U.S. Only mammography

93

HEALTHCARE SERVICE	FOR	COMMENTS
or without clinical breast examination. —*USPSTF, February 2002.* Clinicians should discuss chemoprevention with women at high risk of developing breast cancer and low risk for adverse effects of chemoprevention. —*USPSTF as of December 2003.*		centers with proper accreditation and quality assurance standards should be used. A listing of accredited facilities is available at *www.fda.gov/cdrh/ mammography/certified.html.*
Cervical Cancer Screening (Papanicolaou smear): Women who have a cervix should have a Pap smear at least every three years. Some organizations recommend starting Pap smears for all women who have reached 18 years old, regardless of sexual history. Women over 65 need not be routinely screened if they have had adequate recent screening with normal results and are not otherwise at increased risk for cervical cancer. —*USPSTF,* January 2003 update.	Women within three years of initiation of sexual activity or age 21, whichever comes first	Approximately 16,000 new cases of cervical cancer are diagnosed each year, and about 4,800 women die from this disease annually. The incidence of invasive cervical cancer has decreased over the last 40 years, due in large part to early detection programs.
Colorectal Cancer Screening: The USPSTF strongly recommends that men and women age 50 and older be screened for colorectal cancer. Screening options include home fecal occult blood test, flexible sigmoidoscopy, combination of those, colonoscopy, and	Men and women 50+ who are at average risk. Younger if at high risk.	Colorectal cancer is the fourth most common cancer in the U.S. and the second leading cause of cancer deaths, yet fewer than half of all Americans over 50 are being screened for it. The five-year relative survival rate is over 90% for people whose cancer is found and treated in the early stages of the disease. Less than 30% of cases are detected in an early

HEALTHCARE SERVICE	FOR	COMMENTS
double-contrast barium enema. —*USPSTF, June 2002.*		stage. Most colorectal cancers occur in those at average risk. Those with a family history of colorectal cancer in a first-degree relative have higher risk.
Cardiac Risk Factors		
Tobacco Use: A complete history of tobacco use should be reviewed and intervention for those who use tobacco products should be provided. —*USPSTF as of December 2003.*	All people teens+ and especially pregnant women	Smoking accounts for one out of every five deaths in the U.S. It is the most important modifiable cause of premature death. Major studies provide consistent, convincing evidence linking the use of tobacco with a variety of serious heart diseases and cancers. The majority of all cancers of the lung, trachea, bronchus, larynx, pharynx, oral cavity, and esophagus are attributable to the use of smoked or smokeless tobacco. Smoking also promotes atherosclerosis and is a leading risk factor for heart attacks and coronary artery, cerebrovascular, and peripheral vascular disease. Smoking is also an important risk factor for respiratory illnesses, including chronic obstructive pulmonary disease and pneumonia. Study results vary, but on average, only 22-37% of known smokers who visited a physician or other healthcare professional during the prior year had been advised to quit smoking. Smoking during pregnancy results in the deaths of about 1,000 infants annually. Significant risks associated with smoking during pregnancy include premature births, spontaneous abortions, stillbirths, and intrauterine growth retardation.

HEALTHCARE SERVICE	FOR	COMMENTS
Blood Cholesterol Screening: Routine screening for lipid disorders (abnormal levels of cholesterol in the blood) is recommended. —*USPSTF, March 2001.*	All men 35+ and all women 45+. Men 20-35 and women 20-45, if they have other risk factors for heart disease.	Lipid disorders (high cholesterol) put men and women at risk for heart disease. Heart disease is the leading cause of death in the U.S. Heart attacks kill nearly 500,000 men and women each year.
		Some cholesterol is necessary to maintain cell membranes and other aspects of health. Cholesterol is carried through the blood bound to two types of "lipoproteins." Low-density lipoprotein (LDL) carries most cholesterol in the blood. High levels of LDL can cause clogged arteries. High-density lipoprotein (HDL) helps remove cholesterol from the blood and helps prevent cholesterol buildup. Risk for heart disease increases as levels of LDL increase and levels of HDL decrease. Treatment includes dietary therapy, physical activity, and/or lipid-lowering medications, depending on the patient.
Blood Pressure Screening: The USPSTF recommends blood pressure measurements for patients 21 years or older every two years if their last diastolic and systolic blood pressures were below 85 mm Hg and 140 mm Hg respectively, and annually if their last diastolic was 85–89 mm Hg. —*USPSTF, 1996.* The Seventh Report of the Joint National Committee on Prevention, Detection,	All people 21+	Hypertension (high blood pressure) is a leading risk factor for coronary heart disease, congestive heart failure, stroke, ruptured aortic aneurysm, renal disease, and retinopathy. These complications of hypertension are among the most common and serious diseases in the U.S. Successfully controlling your blood pressure will help you avoid these diseases. Many clinical trials have confirmed the value of controlling blood pressure levels. High blood pressure

HEALTHCARE SERVICE	FOR	COMMENTS
Evaluation, and Treatment of High Blood Pressure new recommendations include: Individuals with a systolic blood pressure of 120-139 mm Hg or a diastolic blood pressure of 80-89 mm Hg should be considered pre-hypertensive and require health-promoting lifestyle modifications to prevent cardiovascular disease. *The JNC 7 Report, May 2003.*		in itself has no symptoms. It is therefore known as a silent killer.
Aspirin for Prevention of Cardiovascular Events: The USPSTF strongly recommends that clinicians discuss the use of aspirin to prevent coronary heart disease with patients who are at increased risk. Potential benefits and harms should be discussed. —*USPSTF, January 2002.*	Men 40+, postmeno-pausal women, younger people with high cholesterol, high blood pressure, diabetes, or a history of smoking	Cardiovascular disease is the leading cause of death in the U.S. The major types of cardiovascular disease are coronary heart disease, which can cause heart attacks, and cerebrovascular disease, which can lead to stroke. Every year, more than 1 million Americans die from heart attacks and other forms of coronary heart disease; nearly 160,000 Americans die from stroke. The USPSTF found good evidence that aspirin decreases the incidence of coronary heart disease (primarily heart attacks) in middle-aged and older adults who are at increased risk but have never had a heart attack or stroke. Data from clinical trials showed that aspirin therapy reduces the risk of coronary heart disease by 28%. Evidence was also found that aspirin increases the incidence of gastrointestinal bleeding and appears to increase slightly the chances of a certain type of stroke.

HEALTHCARE SERVICE	FOR	COMMENTS
Screening for Type 2 Diabetes Mellitus: Screen for impaired glucose tolerance and impaired fasting glucose. —*USPSTF as of December 2003.*	All adults who have high blood pressure or high cholesterol levels	The burden of suffering caused by Type 2 diabetes is enormous. Among individuals aged 40-74, the prevalence increased from 8.9% for the period 1976-1980, to 12.3% for the period 1988-1994. Current prevalence in the United States is likely even higher due to the increasing prevalence of obesity. Patients with Type 2 diabetes are at increased risk of vascular disease, leading to high rates of blindness, end stage renal disease, and lower extremity amputations as well as increased risk for heart disease and stroke. In addition, a substantial number of people who have elevations in blood glucose not meeting criteria for diabetes (impaired fasting glucose or impaired glucose tolerance) are at increased risk for progression to diabetes and for cardiovascular disease.

Preventive Care for Women

Screening for Chlamydial Infection: The USPSTF recommends that all sexually active women age 25 and younger should be routinely screened for chlamydia. —*USPSTF, March 2001.* Women over 25 with new or multiple sexual partners, those in settings where chlamydial infection is common, and those with past sexually transmitted	Sexually active women aged 25 and younger, and women 25+ at high risk	Chlamydia trachomatis is a sexually transmitted infection that affects men and women. It is the most common bacterial sexually transmitted disease in the U.S. Most people who have chlamydia usually do not know it because they have no symptoms. Chlamydia can be treated and cured easily and inexpensively. If not detected, chlamydia can lead to pelvic infection, infertility, and tubal pregnancies. Babies born to women with chlamydia can develop eye infections and

HEALTHCARE SERVICE	FOR	COMMENTS
disease should also be screened. —*USPSTF as of December 2003.*		pneumonia. Women under 25 account for approximately 80% of reported cases. There is a simple urine test now available for detection of this infection.
Screening for Osteoporosis in Postmenopausal Women: Routine screening is recommended. —*USPSTF, September 2002.*	Women 65+ who are at average risk for fractures. Women 60+ who are at high risk for fractures.	Osteoporosis is a condition marked by thinning and weakening of bones and can lead to fractures, loss of height due to compression of the bones in the spine, and pain. Currently, osteoporosis is most commonly diagnosed by finding an abnormal result on x-rays that measure bone mineral density. Fifty percent of all women who live to be 85 years of age will have an osteoporosis-related fracture during their lives; 25% of these women will develop a deformity of the spine, and 15% will fracture a hip. Screening can lead to early detection and treatment, thus preventing fractures.

General Preventive Care

Well Child Care: The American Academy of Pediatrics recommends routine history, physical examination, screening tests, and anticipatory guidance throughout childhood. —*AAP, 1988.*	Children birth-19	Regular well-child checkups are the best way to get your child the preventive care he or she should have. Check *www.preventive services.ahrq.gov* for details on the recommended frequency by child's age.
Well Adult Care: Adults 19-64 should have checkups every one to three years. Those 65 and older should have annual checkups. —*USPSTF, 1989.* No changes to date.	All people 19+	Note that you can safely get checkups every three years instead of every year if you are a basically healthy adult between the ages of 19 and 65, unless you have special risks or needs.

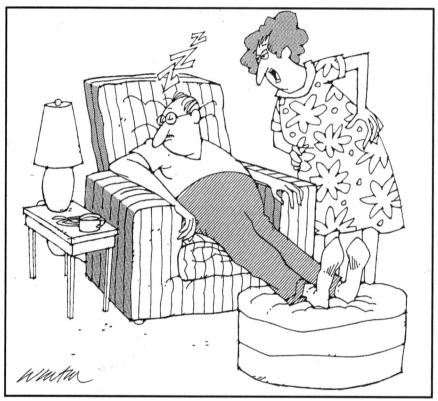

"HOW COULD DR. WILLIS TELL YOU TO SLOW DOWN?"

HEALTHCARE SERVICE	FOR	COMMENTS
Screening for Depression: The USPSTF recommends screening adults for depression in clinical practices that have systems in place to assure accurate diagnosis, effective treatment, and careful follow-up. —*USPSTF, May 2002.*	All adults	Depression is a disabling illness. Between 5% and 9% of adult patients in primary care suffer from depression. Depression increases healthcare utilization and costs $17 billion in lost workdays each year. Despite its high prevalence and its substantial economic impact, depression often goes unrecognized in the primary-care setting. Patients whose depression is undetected cannot be treated appropriately.
Screening for Obesity: All adults should be screened for obesity using Body Mass Index (BMI). A BMI of 30 or higher indicates obesity. Clinicians should provide intensive counseling and behavioral interventions to promote sustained weight loss for obese adults. Effective interventions combine nutrition education and diet and exercise counseling with behavioral counseling to change eating and exercise habits. —*USPSTF as of December 2003.*	All adults	Sixty-one percent of U.S. adults are obese or overweight. 1.7 million Americans die obesity-related deaths every year. Obesity rates have increased by more than 60% among adults in the last 10 years.

Other Advice You Should Receive

The USPSTF also recommends that doctors and other clinicians provide appropriate counseling on the following topics. This list is good for each of us to review to ensure we are taking appropriate preventive measures in each category. The USPSTF would not recommend counseling unless there was good evidence that prevention works in these areas.

Identifying our risk factors, which are based on age, sex, family history, lifestyle, etc., is key to preventing or curbing the onset of disease for each of us.

- Dental and periodontal disease

- Healthful diet (caloric intake control, restriction of fat intake to less than 30% of total calories, limiting cholesterol intake, emphasize foods containing fiber)

- HIV infection

- Household and recreation injuries, including falls (primarily a problem for older persons), poisonings, drownings, fires and burns, mechanical suffocation, choking, firearm injuries, and bicycling injuries

- Motor vehicle injuries (wearing seat belts, avoiding alcohol/drugs when driving)

- Unintended pregnancy

- Structured breastfeeding education and counseling

A Short Summary of Recommended Prevention for "Normal-Risk" Adults

The average adult patient has about a dozen risk factors that require about 24 preventive services.[11] To make it easier to keep track of the basic recommended preventive care, here is a more concise list. Unless you are at high risk for a specific illness, you can use this as a checklist of all the preventive care you need. However, almost everyone is at increased risk for something, based on family or personal history or lifestyle, so don't just assume you are at normal risk for everything. If you are at higher risk than normal for something, you may need to be screened more often or differently. See the chart above and keep checking for updates to screening guidelines based on up-to-date medical research.

For Men

WHAT YOU SHOULD GET	HOW OFTEN	AGES
Screening		
Blood pressure, weight	Periodically	18 years and older
Cholesterol	Every five years	35 years and older
Diabetes	Periodically	Adults with hypertension (high blood pressure) or hyperlipidemia (high cholesterol)
Colorectal cancer	Periodically	50 years and older
Alcohol use	Periodically	18 years and older
Vision and hearing	Periodically	65 years and older
Immunization		
Tetanus-Diptheria	Every 10 years	18 years and older
Varicella	Susceptibles only: two doses	18 years and older
Pneumococcal	One dose	65 years and older
Influenza	Yearly	50 years and older
Chemoprevention		
Discuss with your doctor aspirin to prevent cardio-vascular events	Periodically	40 years and older
Counseling		
Tobacco cessation, drug and alcohol use	Periodically	18 years and older
Sexually transmitted disease and HIV	Periodically	18 years and older
Nutrition, physical activity	Periodically	18 years and older
Sun exposure	Periodically	18 years and older
Oral health	Periodically	18 years and older
Injury prevention	Periodically	18 years and older
Review all over-the-counter, herbal, and prescribed medications taken	Periodically	18 years and older

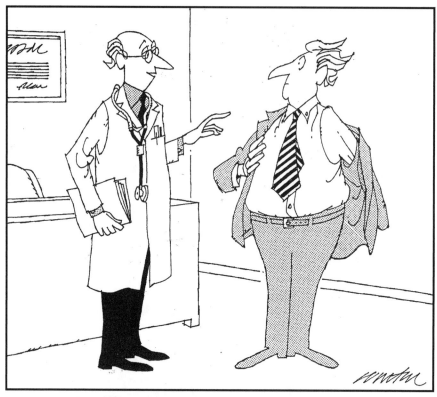

"CUT OUT ALL THOSE LITTLE INTIMATE DINNERS
FOR TWO UNLESS THERE'S SOMEONE WITH YOU."

For Women

WHAT YOU SHOULD GET	HOW OFTEN	AGES
Screening		
Blood pressure, height and weight	Periodically	18 years and older
Cholesterol	Every five years	45 years and older
Diabetes	Periodically	Adults with hypertension (high blood pressure) or hyperlipidemia (high cholesterol)
Pap smear	Every one to three years	18-65 years
Chlamydia	Check with your doctor	18-25 years
Mammography	Every one to two years	40 years and older
Colorectal cancer	Periodically	50 years and older
Osteoporosis	Routinely	65 years or older
Alcohol use	Periodically	18 years and older
Vision and hearing	Periodically	65 years and older
Immunization		
Tetanus-Diptheria	Every 10 years	18 years and older
Varicella	Susceptibles only: two doses	18 years and older
Measles, mumps, rubella	One dose	Women of childbearing age
Pneumococcal	One dose	65 years and older
Influenza	Yearly	50 years and older
Chemoprevention		
Discuss with your doctor aspirin to prevent cardiovascular events	Periodically	50 years and older
Counseling		
Calcium intake	Periodically	18 years and older
Folic acid	Periodically	18-50 years
Tobacco cessation, drug and alcohol use	Periodically	18 years and older
Sexually transmitted disease and HIV	Periodically	18 years and older

Nutrition, physical activity	Periodically	18 years and older
Sun exposure	Periodically	18 years and older
Oral health	Periodically	18 years and older
Injury prevention	Periodically	18 years and older
Review all over-the-counter, herbal, and prescribed medications taken	Periodically	18 years and older

Improving Prevention

Some healthcare organizations have new methods for delivering preventive care. Many have systematized ways of identifying members by age and risk to make sure each member gets the preventive care he or she should have. Find out if your health plan or doctor does this. If you aren't affiliated with a health plan or healthcare organization with this type of outreach, you will need to proactively make sure you are getting every preventive screening or other type of medical preventive service you need.

Help Your Doctor Give You the Preventive Care You Need

Primary-care physicians sometimes forget or neglect to give appropriate preventive care or counseling due to superseding pressures from patients during office visits.[12] For example, if you insist your doctor prescribe medications you don't need, or worse, should not have, your doctor may get so caught up in whether or how to say "No" that he forgets to remind you to get a mammogram.

Doctors often must deal with overriding patient concerns about other issues, patient pressure to prescribe antibiotics they don't need, and other doctor–patient relationship challenges. The lesson here is that you should be careful not to distract your doctor from providing the preventive care you need. In fact, it should be your practice to check in about preventive care schedules with your doctor every time you see him or her.

Ask: "Is My Care On Track?"

A recent commentary by a prominent physician discusses "clinical inertia"—the failure of doctors to stay appropriately in control of therapy for certain types of health problems such as high blood pressure, high cholesterol, and diabetes.[13] Blood pressure level is adequately controlled in only a minority of high blood pressure patients. Only 14-38% of patients with high cholesterol levels are treated to reach appropriate cholesterol levels, and only 33% of patients treated for diabetes reach recommended blood sugar levels. According to this doctor's commentary, "clinical inertia" is due to at least three problems:

- Doctors tend to think the care they have already provided will solve the problem, and then they don't check to make sure this is true.

- Doctors tell themselves that the patient is beginning to make lifestyle improvements that will have a positive impact on the case. They then don't follow up to make sure this is actually happening, ready to step in with other resolutions if not.

- Some doctors may not have the appropriate training or may not have their practices sufficiently well organized to follow up on these escalation-of-care treatments.

No medication can take the place of regular exercise, weight control, not smoking, and eating sensibly.

The lesson here is that YOU must make sure you are checked for high blood pressure, high cholesterol, and diabetes. And YOU must make sure the treatment your doctor has prescribed for these conditions is actually working to reduce the problem. According to the statistics, you can't necessarily rely on your doctor to check this.

In fact, you need to keep tabs on your blood pressure, cholesterol, and blood sugar levels yourself. Inexpensive home blood pressure monitors are widely available (check your local drugstore), and community health fairs offer cholesterol and blood sugar screening tests. Take advantage of these services. If your results show you have a problem or potential problem, take the results to your doctor for advice and treatment.

According to one good study, the prevention services most highly recommended are not provided to patients anywhere near as often as they should be.[14] These are the prevention services that rank highest in terms of disease prevention and cost-effectiveness (cost of the service divided by quality-adjusted life years saved). The highest ranked preventive services with the lowest delivery rates (50% or less nationally) were: providing tobacco cessation counseling to adults, screening older adults for undetected vision impairments, screening adults for colorectal cancer, screening young women for chlamydial infection, screening adults for problem drinking, and vaccinating older adults against pneumonia.

An Ounce of Prevention…Goes a L-o-o-o-ong Way

For your own sake, don't hold onto our society's prevalent "fix-it" mindset. Don't expect a magic bullet—a pill to diminish every one of your risk factors. No medication can take the place of regular exercise, weight control, not smoking, and eating sensibly. Relying on medicine to "fix it" is inviting a preventable disability. No kidding! (More of this lecture in the next chapter!)

The medical system, however, should provide appropriate prevention and screening. And it should provide this for each of us, not just some of us. *Make sure you are getting your fair share of the best, most appropriate, proven, age-specific, gender-specific preventive care that medicine has to offer.*

Pete

This is the story of a man who ignored warning signs for a long time before finally "getting it" and giving himself the chance to live a good life for as long as possible.

Pete is a 60-year-old businessman who, beginning at a very young age, started and managed several highly successful business ventures. Pete dedicated many hours a day to developing and running his businesses. His lifestyle was fast-paced and highly stressful. He ate whatever he could easily grab, often at odd hours, and with little consideration for nutrition. He squeezed in a few games of tennis with a buddy on the odd weekend but otherwise got no real exercise. He had put on a few pounds over the years but did not view himself as having a weight problem.

Pete's first health wake-up call came at age 30, when his 55-year-old father died suddenly of a heart attack. Pete was outraged that his father had died so young and thought his father's doctor should have prevented the heart attack. Eventually, though, Pete convinced himself that his father had just somehow been unlucky. Unlike his father, he was strongly in control of his own destiny, or so he thought.

Pete's second wake-up call came five years later, when his mother died at age 60—also of heart disease. This time, in the midst of Pete's shock and grief, Pete's mother's doctor took him aside for a chat. The doctor pointed out that—with both parents having a history of serious heart disease—Pete should pay attention to his own risk of dying prematurely from the same disease.

Not long after his mother's funeral, Pete began reading about heart disease prevention. He also went to see his mother's doctor to get a checkup for the first time in several years. The doctor arranged for Pete to have some tests to determine the state of his heart's health. As it turned out, Pete's blood cholesterol level was dangerously high, and his blood pressure was also on the high side. The doctor counseled Pete to lose 20 pounds, change his diet, begin getting some regular aerobic exercise, and come back to see him every three months to check his progress.

At first, Pete made definite improvements in his diet—eating more salads and less fast food and decreasing his salt and fat intake. He also started working out three times a week and getting in a regular game of tennis on the weekends. After about a month or so, however, he gradually began drifting back to his old eating patterns and skipping his workouts. Initially losing five pounds, Pete gained all the weight back when he returned to his old behavior.

At his first three-month checkup, Pete's blood pressure was even higher than it had been previously, and there was no change in his cholesterol level. The doctor put him on medications for both. Thinking that the medications would take care of his heart health risks, Pete continued with his old eating patterns and lack of regular exercise. He canceled his second three-month checkup due to a scheduling conflict at work. He did not reschedule the appointment, thinking that the doctor just wanted to earn another payment on his BMW by having Pete make unnecessary office visits.

Fortunately for Pete, he was given a third wake-up call—this one about a year after his mother's death when being screened for new life insurance coverage. He was denied life insurance because both his cholesterol and blood pressure were dangerously high. Pete was shaken to the core. He took a two-week vacation and spent it contemplating the prospect of an early death. He again changed his diet and this time figured out how he could keep himself on the diet by buying specific foods at the grocery store. He asked his friend Linda, with whom he spent a great deal of time, to help him eat more healthfully. She agreed and was helpful in reminding Pete about his commitment to health whenever he began to waver.

Three months after renewing his commitment to health, Pete had lost seven pounds. His doctor told him his cholesterol and blood pressure levels had come down some but not enough. The doctor changed Pete's medications to stronger levels and said it was important both to take the medications regularly and to maintain his new diet and exercise program.

Within six months, Pete's cholesterol and blood pressure had decreased but were still at higher than desirable levels. However, the doctor felt that these levels were about the best Pete could achieve, due to his genetic predisposition to heart problems. He warned Pete that to maintain this acceptable risk level, he would have to maintain his healthy behaviors for the rest of his life.

At age 60, Pete is still alive, though he has begun to suffer some heart disease problems. Pete has maintained his 25-pound weight loss for several years, watches what he eats very carefully, jogs a mile every day, and reads all new information he can find about heart disease prevention and treatment. Pete now understands that he alone must take responsibility for his health. He sees a doctor to make sure he is keeping his health risks as low as possible. He knows that his heart will gradually become less and less healthy as he ages and will probably do so at a more rapid rate than many other people experience, in spite of the preventive measures he takes. However, he also knows that he is doing the best he can do and that what he is doing is keeping him in better health longer.

8 More Benefits of Prevention

Men's natures are alike. It is their habits that carry them far apart.
—Confucius

There are many things we can control that make us less vulnerable to illness. None of them comes in a pill.
—Rachel Naomi Remen, MD[1]

> **In This Chapter...**
> Your daily choices concerning your lifestyle—including diet, exercise, use of alcohol and tobacco, and stress management—have far more impact on your health than any medical care.

A bank robber was asked why he robbed banks. His response: "Because that's where the money is." This chapter is "where the money is" for your health.

I created this chapter separate from Chapter 7 because, although that chapter also discusses prevention, its focus is the preventive services offered by our healthcare system. Here I focus on the prevention measures you and I can and should take for ourselves. Pete's story on the previous pages illustrates how a person can take charge of his or her own life-threatening situation and live as long and disability-free as possible.

Making big changes in how we live day-to-day is not easy. Each of us has to choose how seriously we want to pursue long-term health. The reality is that we probably won't see the major payoffs for making radical health-related lifestyle changes for 30 years or more. Even though we seem to have a national obsession for health information, and we panic when we think we may be denied needed healthcare, we are often not willing to make the tough changes in our behavior that will have the most impact on our health!

Such changes require commitment, energy, and fortitude. For example, it can be really hard to fit into our busy lives the amount of exercise now recommended by the experts. We all tend to wonder if it is really worth it.

The answer is a resounding "Yes." Research shows that avoiding some activities and increasing others *can* help us live longer and with less disability. According to the Institute for the Future, a non-profit research group, research has shown that the following factors, on average, determine our health:[2]

Research shows that avoiding some activities and increasing others *can* help us live longer and with less disability.

Health Behaviors (lifestyle)	50%
Environment	20%
Genetics	20%
Access to Care	10%

This research shows that health-related lifestyle behaviors have far and away more influence on our health than any other factors. In fact, the medical care we get or don't get has the least impact on our health, on average, compared to health-related behaviors, our environment, and our personal genetic structure. Most of us know that eating right, getting adequate exercise, not smoking, and not drinking to excess are good for us. However, my guess is that few of us fully realize how much our choices in these areas affect our health.

The "E" Word and Other Harsh Language

"Opportunity may knock only once. Temptation leans on the doorbell."

— Anonymous

Most of us ignore what we know we should do much of the time. Few people get enough exercise. Most Americans eat pretty unhealthfully much of the time. As health-conscious as I am, even I don't always like taking the time to get the amount of exercise I need—that is, until I remember the health risks I am taking when I don't. I struggle to eat the recommended portions of healthy vegetables every day, and it's very hard for me to stay away from too many sweets, even though I know how important a good diet is for my long-term health.

Franklin-Covey, a highly respected organization that guides other organizations and individuals to greater effectiveness and productivity, recently conducted a nationwide survey to identify "What Matters Most to Americans." The results of the survey showed that "staying physically fit" ranked 8th on the list of life's most important issues, after more important things such as "the health and well-being of my family," "maintaining a close relationship with my family," and so on.

Eighty-four percent of survey respondents said it was important to them to stay physically healthy, and 74% said it was important to take care of their bodies. Yet only 62% believed in the importance of a good diet, and only 47% thought that exercising is important. And, though many people ranked "staying fit" as highly important, personal satisfaction in this area ranked 20th on the list in this same survey, indicating that we are in general not nearly as satisfied with our personal fitness as we would like to be.[3] But if 74% said they want to take care of their bodies, and only 62% believe in the importance of a good diet, and even fewer think it is important to exercise, it seems we are either confused, poorly informed, or we don't want to face the facts.

Now This'll Kill Ya

- Smoking is the number one cause of premature death in the U.S. Lack of physical activity and poor diet, taken together, are the second largest underlying cause of premature death, according to the National Institute on Aging.[4]

- Unhealthy diet and physical inactivity play an important role in many chronic diseases and conditions, including Type 2 diabetes, hypertension, heart disease, stroke, breast cancer, colon cancer, gallbladder disease, and arthritis.[5]

- In 2000, healthcare costs associated with physical inactivity were more than $76 billion.[6]

- Despite the proven benefits of physical activity, more than 60% of American adults do not get enough physical activity to provide health benefits.[7] More than 25% of adults are not active at all.[8]

- Only about one-fourth of U.S. adults eat the recommended five or more servings of fruits and vegetables each day.[9]

- Since 1980, obesity rates have doubled among children and tripled among adolescents. Almost 15% of American children and adolescents are overweight.[10]

So, what specifically do our bodies need?

Most of us ignore what we know we should do much of the time.

Exercise[11]

The benefits of exercise are numerous and great, and the risks associated with not getting adequate exercise are significant. If we face these facts, we've just got to make time to be physically active regularly, no matter what it takes.

- Sedentary behavior (little to no recreational, household, or occupational physical activity) is one of the strongest risk

Become More Active

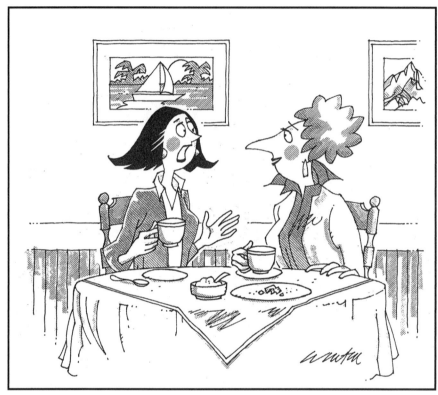

"I'D LOVE TO GO HIKING, BUT HARRY KEEPS FINDING EXCUSES. HIS IDEA OF ROUGHING IT IS BRAN MUFFINS."

factors for many chronic diseases and conditions, including cardiovascular disease, hypertension, diabetes, obesity, osteoporosis, colon cancer, and depression. If you get moderate to vigorous exercise on a regular basis, you can lower your risk of developing these diseases by 30–50%[12].

- People who get an hour a day of very vigorous exercise, either on the job or at leisure, showed a 28% reduced risk of mortality compared with those who got much less exercise, in a recent study conducted by a researcher at the Harvard School of Public Health.[13]
- Exercise helps in weight control, reduces stress, and helps build strong bones, muscles, and joints.

Recent surveys show that:[14]

- Women are less active than men at all ages.
- African Americans and Hispanics are generally less active than whites.
- Adults in northeastern and southern states tend to be less active than adults in north-central and western states.

How Much Exercise Do You Need?

Each of us should have 30 minutes of moderate activity five or more days per week, or 20 minutes of vigorous activity three or more times per week. An hour of moderate activity daily reaps even more health benefits, according to recommendations issued in Fall 2002 by the Institute of Medicine. Moderate-intensity activity refers to any activity that burns three-and-a-half to seven calories per minute. This equates to the effort a healthy individual might burn while walking briskly, mowing the lawn, dancing, swimming for recreation, or bicycling. Vigorous activity burns more than seven calories per minute, such as the effort involved for a healthy individual while jogging, engaging in heavy yard work, doing high-impact aerobic dancing, swimming continuous laps, or bicycling uphill.

Does a Little Exercise Help?

Yes, research shows some benefits for lesser levels of activity, like walking or biking 30 minutes per day on most days of the week. Risk for all causes of death is decreased somewhat by these activity levels, but not as much as for those who get more vigorous exercise on a regular basis.

> Sedentary behavior is one of the strongest risk factors for many chronic diseases and conditions, including cardiovascular disease, hypertension, diabetes, obesity, osteoporosis, colon cancer, and depression.

Eating Right

A report released by the Department of Health and Human Services shows that 61% of U.S. adults are obese or over-weight, and 1.7 million Americans die obesity-related deaths every year.[15] The Centers for Disease Control reports that obesity rates in the U.S. have increased by more than 60% among adults in the last 10 years.[16] The number of overweight and obese U.S. adults is at an all-time high. This is pretty alarming. It reflects the fact that our environment has an overabundance of food—period—and especially foods that are high in saturated fat, low-quality carbohydrates, and sodium.

The sad fact is that this overabundance of unhealthy foods has been increasing. Fast-food and snack food makers have dramatically increased their offerings over the past few de-cades, and the number of fast-food outlets per capita doubled from 1972 to 1997.[17] The competition to capture market share is intense, with new tasty offerings being made every day. It takes serious self-control to not give in to the food temptations all around us. The majority of us apparently are giving in to temptation too often. All age groups, both sexes, and all races are affected.

And note that about 28% of overweight people say their weight is "just about right," while 24% of people who think they are overweight are in fact normal weight or underweight, based on their Body Mass Index.[18]

To calculate your Body Mass Index (BMI), multiply your weight in pounds by 703. Then divide that result by your height in inches squared. A person with a BMI of 25 or higher is overweight. A person with a BMI of at least 50 is consid-ered extremely obese. Ordinary obesity is defined as having a BMI of 30-35. The National Institutes of Health provides a BMI calculator at *www.nhlbisupport.com/bmi* and a table at *www.nhlbi.nih.gov/guidelines/obesity/bmi_tbl.htm*. The Centers for Disease Control and Prevention provides a BMI calculator at *www.cdc.gov/nccdphp/dnpa/bmi/calc-bmi.htm*.

Being overweight puts you at much higher risk for develop-ing metabolic syndrome (also known as pre-diabetes), diabe-tes, heart disease, liver disease, some types of cancer, arthritis, and several other health problems. In recent years there has been a 70% increase in the number of diabetes cases in the U.S. among people 30-39,[19] directly related to the increase in the percentage of people who are overweight and obese.[20] The

> Each of us should have 30 minutes of moderate activity five or more days per week.

increased costs of medical care related to these increases in weight gain will impact each person who has these problems.

The rapid increase in children's obesity is alarming. One of the scariest predictions experts are making is that if we don't get this overweight epidemic under control for our children, "We are going to have the first generation of children who are not going to live as long as their parents."[21]

How Much to Eat Versus What to Eat

It appears from the research outlined above that how much we eat is currently at least as much a problem as what we eat. We need to reduce the total number of calories we consume. It is the intake of more calories than our bodies need that is at the root of the problem.

Regarding what to eat, diseases directly related to unhealthful eating habits are among the leading causes of illness and death in the U.S. Major diet-related diseases include coronary heart disease, some types of cancer, stroke, hypertension, osteoporosis, and Type 2 diabetes.

Also regarding what to eat, there is a lot of confusion about good nutrition these days. Most of us are not nutrition experts. Many snack and fast-food marketers take advantage of our lack of nutritional knowledge, trying to convince us that the food they sell is somehow good for us. Recommendations about how much protein we should eat vary widely among people we might consider experts, adding to our confusion. Experts also disagree about the amount of fat that is healthful to consume. It seems prudent to stick with mainstream research, which suggests the following guidelines:[22]

• Keep serving sizes moderate.

• Eat at least four (4) servings of a variety of vegetables and three (3) servings of a variety of fruits daily. **These foods should constitute the largest volume in your daily diet.** Be sure your fruit and vegetable intake is enough to give you adequate fiber to keep your digestive system functioning properly. One serving of fruit is, for example, one tennis-ball-sized apple.

• Eat four to eight (4-8) servings of carbohydrates daily, emphasizing whole grain breads and cereals. One serving of pasta equals one-half cup; one serving of bread equals one slice.

• Eat three to seven (3-7) servings of protein/dairy daily. Moderate your total fat intake associated with these foods.

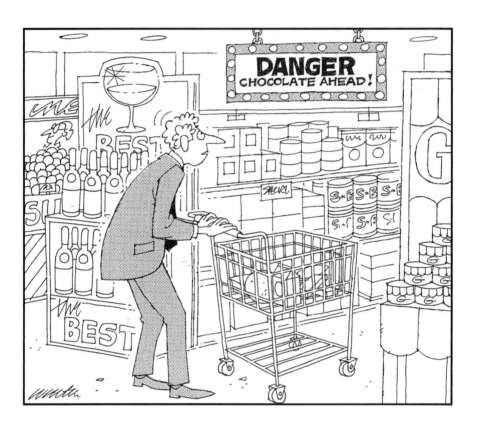

One serving of meat or fish equals two to three (2-3) ounces; one serving of cheese equals one and a half (1.5) ounces.

- Eat three to five (3-5) servings of fat daily, including nuts. Eat mostly unsaturated fats, like olive oil, rather than saturated fats, like butter.

- Limit "empty" (low nutrition) calories, such as sweets, to very small amounts compared to your total food intake. The Mayo Clinic recommends up to 75 calories, which isn't even one big cookie, per day. Sweetened beverages, like sodas, are in this category, too.

> It is the intake of more calories than our bodies need that is at the root of the problem.

If you think about it, these guidelines suggest eating the kind of diet that our prehistoric ancestors would have eaten daily, under the best circumstances of those times. This makes sense because the human body evolved during a time when survival demanded eating the foods that were available. These dietary guidelines suggest staying away from many of the foods that line our supermarket shelves and are so conveniently available in fast-food outlets and restaurants—foods that are highly processed and/or low in the fiber and nutrients we need, many having a lot of empty calories.

Smoking

Twenty-three percent of Americans continue to smoke despite powerful evidence of the risks of using tobacco. Smoking will result in disability and premature death for half of them. Tobacco is the leading cause of preventable death in the U.S.[23]

Statistics on Tobacco Use[24]

- Smoking accounts for one out of every five deaths in the U.S. It is responsible annually for an estimated 5 million years of potential life lost.

- Tobacco is one of the most potent of cancer-causing agents. The majority of all cancers of the lung, trachea, bronchus, larynx, pharynx, oral cavity, and esophagus are caused by use of smoked or smokeless tobacco. Smoking also accounts for a significant percentage of cancers of the pancreas, kidney, bladder, and cervix.

- Smoking promotes atherosclerosis and is a leading risk factor for heart attacks and coronary artery, cerebrovascular, and peripheral vascular disease (in layman's terms: hardening of the arteries, heart attack, stroke).

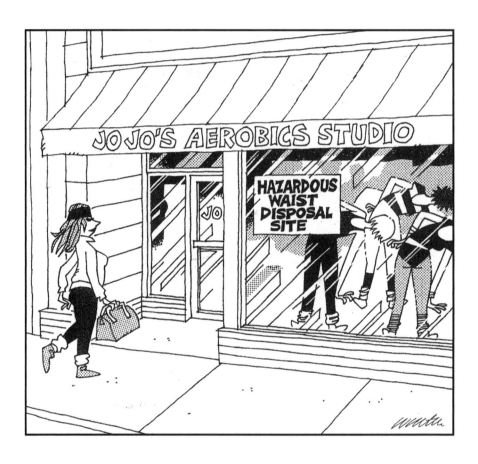

- Smoking is an important risk factor for life-threatening respiratory illnesses such as chronic obstructive pulmonary disease and pneumonia.

- Children and adolescent smokers have increased prevalence and severity of respiratory symptoms and illnesses, decreased physical fitness, and potential retardation of lung growth.

- Nicotine is an addictive drug. The processes that determine nicotine addiction are similar to those that determine addiction to drugs such as heroin and cocaine.

- Starting tobacco use at an early age is associated with more severe addiction as an adult. Most smokers begin smoking as teenagers.

- Smoking affects the health of nonsmokers through inhalation of tobacco smoke.

- Smoking during pregnancy is linked to about 5-6% of perinatal deaths, 17-26% of low-birth-weight births, and 7-10% of preterm deliveries. It increases the risk of miscarriage and fetal growth retardation.

- Many of these health risks can be reduced by stopping smoking. Smokers who quit before age 50 have up to half the risk of dying in the next 15 years that continuing smokers have. After 10 years of abstinence, the risk of lung cancer is 30-50% lower than that of continuing smokers. Risks for other diseases are similarly decreased.

Tobacco is the leading cause of preventable death in the U.S.

What to Do If You Smoke?

You know the answer to this question. Stop. Because nicotine use is an addiction, quitting is not easy. Smokers often start the quitting process multiple times before they are successful. Check with your doctor and health plan to find out what programs are available. There are now medications and sophisticated counseling programs to help you quit.

Drinking

Overuse of alcohol, as we all know, is a health risk. Problem drinking includes more than just the extreme—alcoholism. Many problem drinkers have medical or social problems related to their alcohol use, without typical signs of dependence. All heavy drinkers are putting themselves at risk for future medical problems.

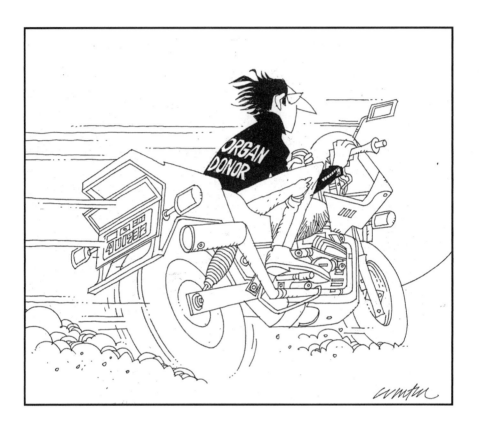

Statistics and Facts

- Medical problems due to alcohol dependence include alcohol withdrawal syndrome, psychosis, hepatitis, cirrhosis, pancreatitis, thiamine deficiency, neuropathy, dementia, and cardiomyopathy.

- Nondependent heavy drinkers account for the majority of alcohol-related illnesses and deaths.

- All causes of alcohol-related deaths have been most closely linked to four or more drinks per day in men and above two drinks per day in women. Their smaller size and slower metabolism cause women to reach higher blood alcohol levels from fewer drinks than men do. Research shows that deaths were 30-38% higher among men and more than double among women who drank six or more drinks per day, compared to nondrinkers and light drinkers.

- Of the more than 100,000 deaths attributed to alcohol use each year, nearly half are due to unintentional and intentional injuries, including traffic fatalities, deaths from fires, drownings, homicides, and suicides.

- People who overuse alcohol have a higher rate of divorce, depression, suicide, domestic violence, unemployment, and poverty.

- Millions of children are at risk for abnormal psychosocial development due to the abuse of alcohol by their parents.

- Excess use of alcohol during pregnancy can produce fetal alcohol syndrome or some of its symptoms, including growth retardation, facial deformities, and nervous system dysfunction.

- Adolescent drinking, especially binge drinking, is directly affiliated with 50% of the leading causes of death in adolescents and young adults: motor vehicle and other unintentional injuries, homicides, and suicides. Frequent binge drinking among young people is also associated with problems keeping up with schoolwork, involvement in unplanned or unsafe sex, and trouble with police.

The Sun and Your Skin

The most common cancer in the U.S. is skin cancer, and the rates for this cancer are increasing. There are three types of skin cancer: melanoma (the most serious), basal cell carcinoma, and squamous cell carcinoma. Projections for 2003 (not yet confirmed) are that approximately 54,200 people contracted melanoma, with 7,600 dying from this disease. Estimates are that about 1 million people developed one of the other two types of skin cancer in 2003.

The best way to prevent skin cancer is to stay out of direct sun exposure or at least wear protective clothing or sunscreen while exposed. Wearing sunscreen tends to make people feel they can stay in the sun longer than they would otherwise, though, and the sunscreen does not fully protect against the longer exposure. It is better to wear protective clothing when in the sun whenever possible, including long sleeves and hats. Those who have a family history of skin cancer, are fair skinned, have red or blonde hair, have a propensity to burn, have an inability to tan, or get greater than average sun exposure are at higher risk and should be checked regularly for skin problems by a knowledgeable doctor.

The Consequences of Risky Behaviors on Health

Riding motorcycles, not using seat belts, engaging in unprotected sexual activity, not getting adequate rest and sleep, and other behaviors also pose health risks. This chapter would not be complete without cautioning you to look at all of your habits and behaviors from a health-risk standpoint and advising you to give serious thought to making changes to lower those risks. Ask yourself if you are sure you are willing to accept the consequences if you become one of the statistics.

Happiness vs. Gratification

Day-to-day happiness has more to do with the pursuit of personal fulfillment than with any pleasure-giving activities we may engage in (eating pastries or drag-strip racing, for example). And though research hasn't proven the link, we all know that a sense of contentment in the mind, body, and soul has a powerful impact on our long-term health. How do you get this sense of fulfillment and contentment? Each of us has to find the answer to that question.

I encountered valuable advice in a recent article titled "Health, Happiness, and the Well-Lived Life: A Doctor's Prescription" by Dr. Rachel Naomi Remen.[25] She suggests we can be happier and more fulfilled by paying closer attention to our true selves. The lifelong process of discovering, exploring, and honoring the best within us is a challenging but potentially immensely satisfying journey.

Part IV

The Elements of Medical Quality

Part IV gives you the signposts of medical quality. Each chapter provides a quick overview of one element of quality of care. Stay with me here. Understanding this information is key to your ability to get the best care. Most consumers lack this knowledge. Without it, it is impossible for you to tell whether or not you are receiving high-quality care.

Sam

Sam is 65. When he began feeling tired much of the time but had no other new symptoms, he assumed this was just part of getting older. However, his tiredness became so severe that he thought he'd better see a doctor about it. Normally he saw a specialist twice a year for arthritis, and he had just seen her two months earlier. He had not seen a primary-care doctor for some time, thinking that seeing the specialist was all he needed to do.

When Sam finally visited a primary-care doctor, the doctor told Sam that he suspected some serious arterial blockage. He sent Sam for lab work and a cardiac catheterization test. The test confirmed a 95% blockage of a major artery. The doctor told Sam that he must have Coronary Artery Bypass Graft (CABG) surgery immediately. The doctor arranged to have the surgery performed by a surgeon he recommended.

Sam's wife, Dorothy, had heard that some hospitals had better survival rates for certain types of surgeries than others. Dorothy called her friend Ellie, who had mentioned this to her, and asked her where she could find out which local hospital was rated best for this specific procedure. Ellie, a retired schoolteacher who is considered a "health nut," collects all kinds of information about health, wellness, and healthcare.

Ellie found the article she had read about the Leapfrog Group. The article gave the website address for this organization, which focuses on hospital quality. She also remembered reading a research report showing that outcomes for certain types of surgeries tended to be better when done in hospitals that do higher volumes of specific types of surgeries and by surgeons who also have done more of these surgeries relative to other surgeons, including CABG surgery. Ellie wanted to help Sam, so she went to the local library and asked the librarian to help her access the Internet and look on the Leapfrog Group website for quality comparison information about the hospitals in the local area. Sure enough, it turned out that one particular local hospital had a higher survival rate for CABG surgery than all the others. Ellie printed the report from the website. She also found and printed the research report about the better outcomes of surgeons with more experience doing certain surgeries.

Ellie dropped by to see Dorothy and Sam that evening and gave them the reports. Since Sam's surgery was scheduled in a hospital that was not the best on the list, Sam angrily called his doctor the next morning and told him he wanted his surgery done in the best hospital and by a doctor who had done a large number of CABG surgeries with generally good outcomes. The doctor tried to talk Sam out of this notion, saying that the hospital ratings were questionable. He said that the hospital where Sam's surgery was scheduled was a good one, as was the surgeon he recommended, even though neither the hospital nor the surgeon had done a comparatively high volume of this type of surgery. However, the information from Ellie had convinced Sam that he needed to insist on the right hospital and surgeon. And once Sam is committed to an idea, he stubbornly sticks to it! The doctor finally reluctantly agreed to find a surgeon who had done a large number of these surgeries successfully and who did the surgeries at the recommended hospital.

Sam's doctor called him back about an hour later and referred him to a surgeon who had successfully done a large number of CABG surgeries and who would do the surgery at the best hospital, which was where he normally did his surgeries. Sam was enormously relieved. Ellie had also recommended that Sam get as much information about his condition as possible so he could understand what was happening to his body as well as what the surgery would do. She recommended specific, trustworthy websites where he could find the information he needed.

When Sam had spoken with his doctor about rescheduling the surgery, he had also asked him about getting more information about his disease. The doctor agreed that Sam should have as much information as possible, but said that unfortunately there was never enough time in office visits to explain everything. He said that the two websites Ellie had mentioned were well respected for their accuracy, and he agreed that Sam should get the information about his condition from those websites, and then if Sam had questions they could discuss them. So Sam and Dorothy spent the afternoon getting information about his condition from the recommended websites.

By the next morning, Sam and Dorothy had a list of unanswered questions that came up as they were reading the information. Some of the questions had to do with how the information applied exactly to Sam's case. When Sam visited the new surgeon for preparation the day before his surgery, he asked the surgeon his questions. The surgeon was impressed with the research Sam had done. He told Sam he always found that patients who learned as much as possible about their condition and surgery tended to do better than those who did not.

The night before his surgery, Sam was anxious, but he knew that he was less anxious than he would have been if Ellie had not helped find the best hospital and surgeon and if he had not done the research on his condition and gotten his questions answered. He felt somehow more in control than when he first learned about his heart problem.

Sam came through the surgery well and then spent several weeks recuperating at home after spending a week in the hospital. After his surgery experience, he is now much more aware that everyone should check on quality comparison data for all of their healthcare providers.

9 Measuring Healthcare Quality

Teach a highly educated person that it is not a disgrace to fail and that he must analyze every failure in order to find its cause. He must learn how to fail intelligently, for failing is one of the greatest arts in the world. —Charles F. Kettering

---

In This Chapter...
- How and why healthcare quality is measured.
- Using failure as a basis for making improvements.
- How patient satisfaction is measured.
- Problems in measuring quality and patient satisfaction.
- Who does this measuring?

Sam's story illustrates the value of carefully measuring and comparing the outcomes of healthcare under varying situations so we can learn which type of care and circumstances produce the best results. The Leapfrog Group's hospital quality comparison data, which Sam used, gives the same results as the best of several recent research studies. This research shows that surgery done in hospitals and by surgeons with the most experience doing a specific type of surgery has the best average outcomes for the patient. Had this research comparing results of hospitals and surgeons not been done, or if Sam had not found out about it, Sam would not have had any guidance about which hospital and surgeon to use. He would simply have had to trust his doctor to make recommendations. As it turned out in this case, that would not have given Sam the best chance for a good outcome.

We buy airline tickets to get to a destination. We buy exercise equipment or a gym membership to lose weight or become more fit. Similarly, we buy healthcare to remain as healthy as possible and to recover our health when ill. To determine which physicians, hospitals, and health plans offer what we are looking for, we must find out which ones consistently provide patients with the best *results*.

Keeping Score

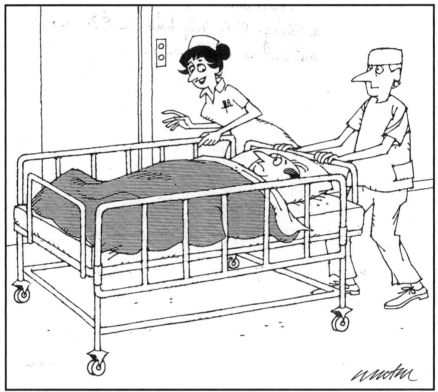

"DON'T WORRY ABOUT A THING. WE ONLY HAVE A
5% ERROR RATE HERE AT MEMORIAL."

Substitute Measures

Results—or "outcomes" as the medical industry refers to them—are the best evidence for quality. And though this is the most logical place from which to assess quality, measuring and comparing actual health outcomes is often extremely difficult. One reason is that true and final results often take years to determine. For this and other reasons, the medical industry often looks at substitute measures for its assessments of quality.

Using substitute measures could be compared to relying on circumstantial evidence in a criminal trial where there aren't any eyewitness accounts. For example, good evidence shows that Pap smears are useful in detecting cervical cancer in its early, treatable stages. Therefore, measuring the number of women who receive Pap smears is a good substitute measure for how well a healthcare system or health plan prevents death from cervical cancer.

Another way to say this is that in medical care "outcome" data may not be available, but data on care processes likely linked to good outcomes may be available. Therefore, the higher the percentage of women receiving Pap smears at the appropriate intervals, the higher the quality of care is deemed to be. But keep in mind that receiving a Pap smear is not a direct measure of survival of cervical cancer. It is a substitute measure of a process that is linked to higher survival rates.

When actual results are not available or are too hard to get, measuring the application of medical care processes is our best way to compare quality of care. When you know that in one health plan, 76% of its female members over 40 have received a Pap smear in the last two years, and in another health plan, 86% of its female members over 40 have received a Pap in the last two years, you know that the second health plan most likely does a better job of catching cervical cancer in its early treatable stages. Therefore, in the category of cervical cancer treatment, the second plan is considered the higher-quality health plan.

The Importance of Measurements

The importance of measuring results of healthcare is twofold:

1. **For consumer information:** To give valid information to healthcare consumers so they can compare the quality of different healthcare sources—to assist them in their healthcare purchasing decisions.

2. **For quality improvement:** To create a baseline of information so each participating physician, hospital, and health plan can make improvements. The provider must know his/her/its level of quality in order to determine what and how much improvement is needed.

Consumer Information

We all want to make wise choices for ourselves and our families, especially when it comes to something as important as health. But without having valid measurements of comparable results (or processes assumed to lead to desired results, as we've seen above), how can we know which physicians, hospitals, and health plans are the best? Most of us have been making judgments in the dark.

Valid quality comparison measurements have not been available until fairly recently. Even now, little information is available comparing the quality provided by individual doctors, though more data becomes available each year. Few consumers are aware that this information exists even in the limited number of areas of the country where it is available. By using valid comparisons, you can make more informed choices.

If most people were receiving good care, then this issue would not be so important. But the evidence indicates that many people get mediocre or even poor care. Therefore, we need to be able to distinguish the high-quality providers from the rest.

Compare buying healthcare with buying a car. The wise shopper, about to make a major investment, researches and compares more than one make and model of car before making a decision. The wise shopper consults third-party quality assessments, such as those found in *Consumer Reports,* as part of his or her research.

Applying the same process to buying healthcare, we should be able to research the quality of a doctor's work before buying his or her services. The same goes for medical groups (groups of doctors working together), hospitals, and health plans. My hope is that, soon, more of this kind of information will become available in all parts of the country and that more people will become aware that it is out there.

Quality Improvement

Feedback is essential for improvement. It's absolutely necessary for making adjustments. If a person (in this case a physician) doesn't know how good or bad his or her work is, he or she can't know in what ways or how much to improve. This is true for you and me in *our* work as well as for physicians, hospitals, and health plans in *their* work.

Performance assessments are commonplace for employees—their salaries and promotions are based upon these evaluations. Athletes measure their running time or their victories or the number of errors they make to assess how they can improve their game. Unfortunately, many healthcare organizations, including physicians, physician groups, health plans, and hospitals, have not yet seriously adopted useful, effective measurement and feedback systems. Therefore, they are unable to see where and how they can improve.

Measuring by Fatalities

A patient either lives or dies during or immediately after surgery, so it is easy to measure a hospital's survival rate for a specific type of surgery. Some surgeries are so risky that measuring their survival rates makes sense. For example, Coronary Artery Bypass Graft (CABG) surgery is a high-risk procedure. Some states require hospitals to report to the state government the mortality (death) statistics for this and other types of high-risk surgeries. In some states, the statistics are publicly available, so consumers can compare results from different hospitals. In other areas, mortality statistics for high-risk procedures may be available from other sources.

Appendix B tells you how to find statistics for hospitals in your area. If you or a family member is scheduled for a high-risk surgery, check all available comparison studies to find the hospital in your area with the best results for that specific procedure. (Please note: Beware of "best hospital" reports based on financial measures—that is, how well each hospital is run financially—rather than medical/surgical measures. These financial analysis reports could be useful to you if you were considering investing in a hospital or hospital system, but will not help you determine whether or not to have surgery there.)

Unfortunately, there isn't much data available on treatments that are not a matter of life or death. Other than knowing if the patients lived, it is difficult to find out how they fared after a particular treatment.

Measuring Nonfatal Results

One or both of the following methods may be used for measuring nonfatal outcomes from procedures. Both require time-consuming and costly action.

> To determine which physicians, hospitals, and health plans offer what we are looking for, we must find out which ones consistently provide patients with the best results.

Measuring Quality

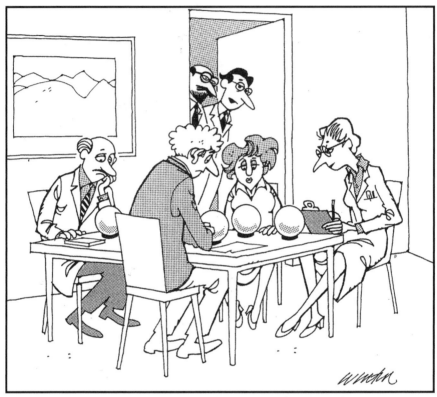

"WE CAN'T FIGURE OUT WHY OUR HEART TRANS-
PLANT PATIENTS KEEP DYING. IF WE CAN'T FIGURE
OUT SOMETHING SOON, WE MAY HAVE TO CHECK
THE PATIENT CHARTS."

- Patients and/or their doctors complete detailed questionnaires about the patient's pain levels and ability to perform normal daily functions after treatment. The responses are then reviewed for completeness and accuracy. Any missing or unclear responses are followed up with the patient or physician who completed the questionnaire. Though the subjective nature of these responses must be taken into account, this is one way to track and compare levels of health and recovery after treatment.

- Alternately, third-party researchers review medical charts to get outcome data. However, the charts often lack detailed information on the patient's ability to perform daily functions. Therefore, though easier than the first, this method yields more limited results.

Both methods require someone to enter the results into a database. Then someone must create meaningful comparison reports from the accumulated data. In these times of dramatically rising healthcare costs, many healthcare organizations have difficulty justifying the expense of data collection and analysis. Additionally, the healthcare industry has not yet established a universally accepted standard for measuring and comparing results for nonfatal treatments.

These excuses are understandable and, to many healthcare executives, very real. Nevertheless, the healthcare organizations that have made the most progress in quality improvement have adopted some means of measuring results. They consider it a worthwhile investment, and it is. If consumers demand data on results of care (or processes of care linked to results) from every health plan or care system, and if consumers refuse to use providers that do not make comparative quality information available, more doctors and hospitals will invest in measurement systems. This will also spur more doctors and hospitals to actually improve the quality of the care they provide.

Risk Adjustment: An Important Factor

To be fair, the measurements of some quality outcomes—such as surgery survival rates—need to be adjusted for the fact that some providers treat sicker patients than others. Sicker patients require even higher-quality care and/or more or different resources than less-ill patients to achieve the same results, and some may have poor outcomes no matter how good the care.

To account for these differences, analysts use "risk-adjustment calculations." They review patients' charts and assign each patient a risk level based on the severity of his or her illness before medical intervention. Then they adjust the results of each patient's outcome relative to his or her initial level of risk.

For example, a patient who was on the brink of death before treatment and who survives a liver-transplant will score higher than a mildly ill patient who survives the same surgery. This type of risk adjustment makes it possible for the outcomes of **higher-risk** patients to be more fairly compared with those of **lower-risk** patients.

Who's Watching the Doctors, Hospitals, and Health Plans?

See Appendix B for sources of comparison data on health plans, medical groups, physicians, and hospitals. One of the main organizations on this list is the National Committee for Quality Assurance (NCQA), a private, non-profit agency that accredits managed care plans (HMOs, POS plans, and PPOs) on a voluntary basis. NCQA rates plans based on a star rating system, with five stars representing the highest rating for HMOs and four stars representing the highest rating for PPOs. Accreditation is based on demonstrated levels of service to members and on clinical quality. See health plan ratings at the NCQA consumer website, *www.healthchoices.org*.

The Joint Commission on Accreditation of Healthcare Organizations (JCAHO, known as "Jayco") is another useful watchdog. This independent, non-profit organization evaluates the quality and safety of care for more than 16,000 health-care organizations. JCAHO standards are considered by many to set the bar for quality of care, especially in hospitals.

Though hospitals were JCAHO's first targets when it was established 50 years ago, it now also evaluates health plans, ambulatory care organizations of many types, assisted living facilities, nursing homes, home care organizations, laboratories, etc. JCAHO's goal is "To continuously improve the safety and quality of care provided to the public through the provision of healthcare accreditation and related services that support performance improvement in healthcare organizations." You can see a list of JCAHO-accredited healthcare organizations and their survey results in JCAHO's Quality Check section online at *www.jcaho.org*, or call their customer service department at 630-792-5800.

In the last few years, new public watchdogs have emerged due to growing concern about widespread poor-quality care that continues despite traditional accreditation processes. The Leapfrog Group now has publicly available quality comparison data on hospitals: *www.leapfroggroup.org*. The National Quality Forum is a non-profit organization charged with developing nationally accepted quality measures. See their website at *www.nqf.org* for a recently-released set of measures for hospitals. Check with your hospital to see if it uses this list of measures of quality as its standards. Most importantly, does your hospital publicly release the data about how it compares in quality measures? If not, you should demand that it do this.

> By using valid comparisons, you can make more informed choices.

HEDIS, the First Useful Quality-Comparison Tool

HEDIS, the Health Plan Employer Data Information Set, is a quality-of-care measurement tool created in the early 1990s by a coalition of health plans and employers. It was designed to gather and compare quality-of-care information that is uniform and consistent for all health plans.

Before HEDIS, health plans reported quality statistics any way they wanted, and there was no way to compare plans in any reliable, consistent manner. Health plans participating in HEDIS surveys report their quality measurements annually to the National Committee for Quality Assurance (NCQA). A comparison report is generated each year.

HEDIS measurements are almost exclusively process measurements, not results measurements, but the process measurements used are closely linked with desired results. Critics feel that HEDIS does not go far enough in measuring quality. This is no doubt true. However, HEDIS measurements are the best data currently available for reliably comparing one health plan to another. HEDIS reports are used in the health-plan ratings provided through NCQA and can be reviewed at the NCQA consumer website, *www.healthchoices.org*.

Measuring Member Satisfaction

Healthcare quality includes more than just the technical aspects of care. Research by the federal Agency for Healthcare Research and Quality identified the non-technical aspects of healthcare that consumers most care about. These include communication, timeliness, responsiveness, and ease of access to services. In recognition of this, now included in HEDIS is a member-satisfaction survey called CAHPS (the Consumer Assessment of Health Plans Survey).

CAHPS includes questions for consumers about whether their health plan gives them access to the care and services they need, whether the health plan resolves grievances quickly and fairly, and how quickly they can get healthcare appointments. Health plans that are rated by NCQA must have a certain number of members complete CAHPS each year. You can review the results of the survey for rated plans at the NCQA consumer website shown above.

Scrutiny Produces Improvement

As more people learn about the quality gaps in American medicine, more attention is focused on fixing the problems. Over the last several years I have seen fast-growing discussion and action on these issues within the healthcare and medical industries. As I write this book I have to constantly check to make sure I have included the most up-to-date information about ways in which quality is being measured. Watch for new and ideally better sources of valid information and quality-promoting activities over the next few years.

10 Evidence-Based Medicine

The saddest aspect of life right now is that science gathers knowledge faster than society gathers wisdom.   —Isaac Asimov

In This Chapter...
- Space shuttle example shows how faulty assumptions can mask the need to gather solid evidence.
- Many physicians are not able to keep up with the overwhelming amount of new information that continuously comes from medical research.
- Medical care of the highest quality uses scientifically proven treatments with solid evidence of effectiveness, but knowledge of and use of these treatments is not widespread.

A Space Age Example

On January 28, 1986, the *Challenger* space shuttle blew up shortly after launch, killing all seven astronauts aboard. As you may remember, the *Challenger* project was known as the "teacher in space" mission because of the inclusion of Christa McAuliffe, an elementary school teacher from New Hampshire. The explosion at launch and the death of the seven crew members, including Ms. McAuliffe, was caused by the failure of O-rings, rubber-like parts designed to seal gaps created by pressure at ignition in the joints of the solid rocket boosters.

Diane Vaughan, a Boston College sociologist, extensively studied the *Challenger* incident and wrote about it in her monumental book, *The Challenger Launch Decision: Risky Technology, Culture, and Deviance at NASA.*[1] The evidence she presents shows that space-program engineers and managers had for years routinely accepted as fact some dangerous, faulty assumptions—which ultimately led to the disaster. Blaming any individual or set of individuals for their actions or inactions misses the point that acceptance of the problematic data had been going on for a long time and had become so routine that it was not recognized as a problem.

Best Available Assumption vs. Hard Data

The pattern of accepting the best available assumptions instead of actually testing to verify data started in NASA's early years, apparently due to cost and performance pressures. As time went on and pressures to perform continued, acceptance of the risky data became a built-in part of the culture of NASA and of its subcontractors.

NASA engineers had noticed damage to O-rings on previous shuttle flights, but because of the pattern of relying on the original assumptions about O-ring tolerances, engineers repeatedly ignored the warning signs. Not until disaster struck did they realize they should have seen the pattern of damage as unacceptable, that their decisions had been based on faulty assumptions, and that further testing of the O-rings should have been conducted long before.

Sadly, the recent loss of the space shuttle *Columbia* and its seven astronauts, 17 years after the *Challenger* incident, was due to a similar pattern of behavior at NASA, according to a report issued by an official investigation team in August 2003. It appears that time and money pressures again led the engineers to take too much risk. Once again, accepting unproven assumptions led to disaster.

Applying Lessons Learned to Medical Treatment

Use these space shuttle disasters as examples of what not to do. Consumers and physicians both need to better understand the pattern of problems in healthcare. We all need to start thinking differently and to stop accepting unnecessary risk.

Just like the space-program engineers, many of our doctors do not know for sure whether the treatments they prescribe actually work as intended. They don't know because either adequate testing has not been done, or they are unaware of existing scientific evidence proving or disproving the value of the treatment.

Medical decisions must be made, just as the decision had to be made about whether to launch *Challenger* on that exceptionally cold January morning. In the *Challenger* decision, the engineers did not realize or acknowledge that there were gaps in their understanding of how the O-rings worked. Faced with pressures to launch, they ultimately made the recommendation to go ahead with the launch based on faulty assumptions.

> An estimated 70% of medical care in the U.S. has never been scientifically confirmed to be the most effective.

But they did not consciously choose to take what turned out to be a huge risk. They thought they were doing the right thing.

Many doctors base their decisions about treatment on assumptions that are just as questionable. In the same way, they are not consciously choosing to put their patients at risk or to provide questionable care. They have to make decisions. Like the NASA managers and engineers, they believe they are doing the right thing. However, only physicians who are keeping up with the latest scientific evidence of what works best can have greater confidence that they ARE doing the right thing.

Most suboptimal medical care is not life-threatening, even if it doesn't accomplish what was intended or doesn't accomplish it in the most effective way. At best, we are spending far more than necessary when we pay for ineffective care. At worst, ineffective treatments put us at risk due to potential side effects.

When no scientific studies exist to guide them in their decision-making, physicians must use the best evidence available at the time. But when there *is* scientific evidence supporting a specific protocol, we should be getting that treatment instead of other, less effective care. Doctors need to at least acknowledge when they are basing their decisions on unproven assumptions and avoid taking unnecessary and inappropriate risks with unproven treatments.

An estimated 70% of medical care in the U.S. has never been scientifically confirmed to be the most effective. To determine which treatments actually work—or which ones work better than others—studies must be carefully designed and controlled. Medical research is constantly updating best practices. Following is a comparison of the old and the new ways of treating patients.

The Old Way: "What I Learned in School"

Traditionally, medical care has relied heavily on the patient's trust in the doctor's compassion and healing abilities. Medical schools trained physicians to administer treatments based on scientific evidence available at the time. But, after graduation, as new information becomes available at an ever-increasing rate, many doctors find it impossible to keep up. By default, doctors may rely on what they learned in medical school—however long ago that was. Until recently, new information was available generally in one of four ways:

• **Professional reading:** Doctors had time to read only a small portion of the vast amount of medical information avail-

Keeping Up with Medical Research

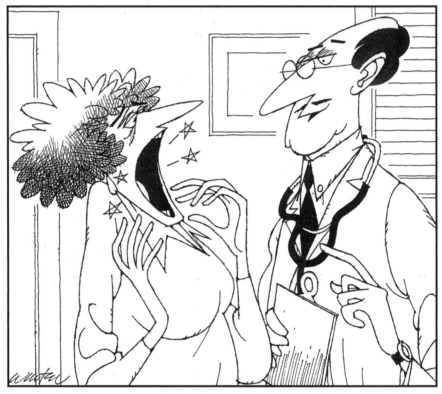

"OOPS! GUESS THAT DIDN'T WORK. I'D BETTER READ UP
ON THIS. I'LL GET BACK TO YOU NEXT WEEK."

able through journals, research findings, and other sources of professional development.

• **Vendor data:** Drug company salespeople provided information on new treatments involving the drugs they sold. (Obviously, this source of data is self-serving and probably biased.)

• **Hallway chats:** Conversations with professional colleagues rounded out the physician's knowledge base.

• **Expert consensus:** When a physician found the time to research the latest options for treatment of a specific diagnosis, the most common approach was to determine who the preeminent experts were considered to be in a given medical specialty area and to find out what treatments those experts favored. However, the "experts" did not always use valid scientific evidence to determine the treatments they used, so "expert opinion" was not a scientifically proven approach to care.

Unfortunately, many U.S. physicians still use these outmoded approaches. A good deal of research on best practices shows that only 30-50% of U.S. physicians use up-to-date treatments.[2] Equally unfortunate is that consumers assume that their doctor knows and uses the best medical practices. All too often, consumers rely far more on blind trust or personality when choosing and working with a physician than on any valid evidence that he or she provides high-quality medical care.

The New Way: "Show Me the Evidence"

Medicine has changed drastically over the last several years. The highest-quality medical care is now based more on up-to-date scientific evidence than ever before. Carefully designed, controlled, and peer-reviewed research is used to find the most successful methods of diagnosis, prevention, and treatment of specific maladies. Previous assumptions are constantly replaced by new and better knowledge. Guidelines for clinical practice are developed based on the results of the new research.

As mentioned above, only about 30% of everyday medical care has current, scientifically determined guidelines available for doctors to use in their treatment decisions,[3] though ongoing medical research continually adds to the knowledge base. In 1983, only 15% of day-to-day medical care had valid, up-to-date scientific evidence to justify it.[4] Science-based guidelines are now available for many of the most common diagnoses.

The Agency for Healthcare Research and Quality (AHRQ) serves as a clearinghouse, publishing on their website (*www.guideline.gov*) up-to-date guidelines developed by credible organizations. The mission of this federal agency is to provide medical research data to improve healthcare quality; enhance patient outcomes; and foster safe, effective, and cost-effective care.

When guidelines are available for a specific illness, physicians who aim to provide high-quality care use them to make treatment decisions. This is called "evidence-based" medicine.

The explosion of medical information over the past few decades has far exceeded doctors' capacity to absorb, let alone apply, all the knowledge every day without some assistance. Doctors need reminder systems and other tools to help them incorporate the latest guidelines into their practices. Today, most doctors do not have these tools and thus are challenged in staying current.

Patients wanting the highest-quality care should look up the guideline data for their diagnosis on the AHRQ website (*www.guideline.gov*) to see what treatment has worked best in clinical trials or other research. If your doctor is aware of the latest guidelines for your symptoms/diagnosis, he or she may have good reasons for varying from the research results in your particular situation, but should be willing to discuss those reasons with you. In any case, use the research data as the basis for a discussion with your doctor. Doing this benefits you in three ways:

1. It ensures that your doctor is aware of the latest medical research on treatments for your diagnosis.

2. It helps you make sure you are getting the best possible care.

3. It helps you form a partnership with your doctor to make decisions about your care.

The following story illustrates the fact that there can be multiple science-based medical "guidelines" that seem to conflict with one another. In many cases the multiple guidelines have been developed by different well-respected medical organizations based on differing interpretations of the same data. This makes it challenging for doctors to determine which variation of the guideline to use. However, using some variation of any guideline is far better than ignoring science-based guidelines altogether.

Mary is 43 and works for a large public agency. She and her husband live in San Francisco. Her employer sends out a monthly employee newsletter, and for the last year or so it has included a Health column that gives tips on wellness. Mary has always been pretty healthy and rarely goes to the doctor except for her well-woman visits to the gynecologist. She is fairly good about making a well-woman appointment every year or so. In one of the recent employee newsletters the Health column mentioned that the American Cancer Society recommends a mammogram every year for women over 40. Mary became concerned that her gynecologist had told her to get a mammogram three years ago but not since. Her annual exam was about due, so she decided to make the appointment as soon as possible and to ask her doctor why he did not tell her to get a mammogram each of the past two years.

At Mary's appointment she discussed this concern with her doctor, and he told her that the results of the medical research done on the value of annual mammography for women 40-49 were unclear. Different organizations interpreted the same data in different ways. Although the American Cancer Society recommended annual mammography for all women 40-49, other respected consensus panels have been unable to agree on the advisability of this recommendation. Instead, a federal panel as well as other highly respected medical organizations recommended that the decision about how often mammograms should be done for this age group should be left to the discretion of physicians and their patients. Mary's doctor's professional opinion, based on reading many scientific articles on the topic, was that women 40-49 with no breast cancer symptoms and who do not have any close family history of the disease should have a mammogram once every three years, not every year.

Mary's doctor had thoroughly discussed Mary's family medical history with her when she first became his patient five years ago. Mary had said at that time that no close relatives on either her mother's or her father's side of the family had had breast cancer. Based on this and other information, he felt that Mary was not at high risk of developing the disease, so she did not need an annual mammogram. He would continue to give her an annual breast exam, and he encouraged her to do regular breast exams

The explosion of medical information over the past few decades has far exceeded doctors' capacity to absorb, let alone apply, all the knowledge every day without some assistance.

You must see to it on your own that your doctor is using the latest medical research as a basis for making treatment decisions.

at home. If she noticed any symptoms she should let him know. Without any indication of symptoms or risk, he felt strongly that to get a mammogram annually at her age was not only an unnecessary hassle and expense, but also has potential risk from false positive results. When mammograms falsely indicate a malignancy (false-positive results are not rare in this age range), they can lead to unnecessary biopsies and the risk of ensuing complications. He even gave Mary a copy of an article by a prominent gynecologist that had been published in a respected medical journal about this issue, promoting the concept of using discretion based on an assessment of risk in determining how often women 40-49 should have mammograms.

It is important to understand that guidelines are often targeted to the average person. Each person's situation may differ. Another key to understanding why guidelines for the same diagnosis differ, based on interpretations of the same scientific data, is that values differ among various medical organizations. For example, with the mammography guidelines for women 40-49, the American Cancer Society believes in screening to reduce cancer deaths and puts less emphasis on the potential side effects of mammography, such as the risks associated with false positives. Guidelines from other organizations, using the same data, place more emphasis on the harms of the screening tests and try to balance the potential benefits and risks. In the case of mammography, some organizations believe that the risks of breast cancer in the 40-49 age category are low enough, and the potential harms of mammography high enough, that recommending annual mammograms is not warranted. So, discussing with your doctor what your values are regarding potential risks and benefits can help determine if breast cancer screening is right for you.

In general, Mary did not want to worry about her health or take unnecessary risks when it did not seem warranted, so she felt the issue was resolved. She was frankly glad not to have to go to the trouble of making the appointment and taking time from work to get a mammogram each year. But she was glad she had asked her doctor about it, and she was glad that he had taken the time to give her a thorough explanation. Mary felt that the explanation her doctor had given her showed that he was on top of the latest medical knowledge. However, just to make sure, Mary spent some time that evening looking up information about mammograms on the Web. The information she found confirmed that there was controversy about how often women in her age bracket should have mammograms. However, she also found that it was true that some highly respected, trustworthy organizations recommended exactly what her doctor recommended. In the end, she decided that the only thing she wished had happened differently is that her doctor had discussed this proactively with her two or three years ago.

Where to Find Good Information on the Web

MedlinePlus (find it at *www.nlm.nih.gov*) is an excellent section on the National Library of Medicine's website that provides well-researched overviews to just about any medical topic you may be looking for, all in consumer-friendly language. The site is constantly updated to reflect the latest scientifically-proven treatment guidelines for specific diagnoses and will also give good information about multiple guidelines for the same diagnosis or treatment. You may find as much information about your diagnosis or other medical issue as you need here, and the site also provides links to other good sources of information.

Don't Confuse Guidelines With Research Studies

Guidelines for the treatment of specific diagnoses are developed by studying the results of many clinical trials. If all of the clinical trials being reviewed have been well designed and therefore produce trustworthy results, and if the results of all or at least most of the trials are approximately the same, it becomes easy to develop a guideline based on all of the clinical trials reviewed.

Let's say, for example, that there have been 30 recent well-structured clinical trials that all show that Pap smears effectively detect cervical cancer in its early stages in 99% of low-risk women over 40 when done every three years just as well as when done every year. This would make it easy to develop a guideline that tells all physicians (and all women) that it is safe to do Pap smears once every three years instead of every year, unless indications exist that the woman is high-risk or unless specific symptoms arise.

Most of the time, however, clinical trials looking at the value of a specific treatment or screening test have a range of

Get the Best Care

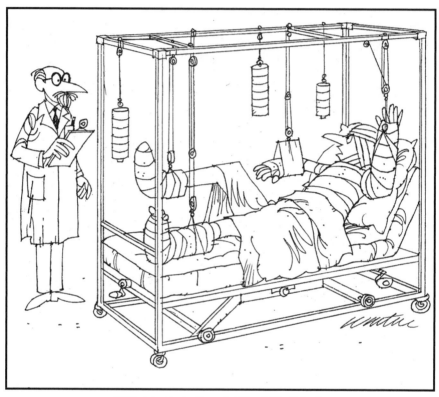

**"I'D LIKE A SECOND OPINION,
FROM A STRUCTURAL ENGINEER."**

results and require careful review by well-trained scientists to sort out the story told by the combination of results. This makes the work of developing a guideline very challenging.

Very often we hear in the news the results of a specific medical research study. It is easy to assume, based on how results are often reported, that the results of that one study should change the way every doctor treats the diagnosis in question. But to the contrary, guideline development should be based on the results of multiple, well-designed studies, unless the one study is extremely large and very carefully designed to give conclusive results.

The National Institute on Aging (NIA) has published a good article explaining what aspects of news reports on medical research studies to look for and what questions to ask as you read the report to better understand the implications of the study results. As of this book's print date, you can get a free copy of this NIA article by going to *www.niapublications.org.* At this website, type the words "Understanding Risk" in the Search box, then click "Search." You will then be guided to order a free copy of "Understanding Risk: What Do Headlines Really Mean?" to be mailed to you.

Ask Your Doctor, "Do You Use Guidelines?"

In Chapter 9, I discussed how HEDIS is being used by the National Committee for Quality Assurance (NCQA) to evaluate health plans. (Remember, HEDIS is an annual survey of how well each participating health plan is doing on certain quality measures.) In fact, most of the HEDIS measures, such as what percentage of women members over 50 receive mammograms, come directly from evidence-based guidelines available on the Agency for Healthcare Research and Quality (AHRQ) website (*www.ahrq.gov* or *www.guideline.gov*).

By choosing a health plan that is highly rated in the NCQA assessment system, you have a better chance of finding a doctor who uses validated guidelines. However, even some doctors who are affiliated with the highest-rated plans don't always use these guidelines. If you look closely at the HEDIS results, you will note that no health plan shows 100% compliance with any guideline. Therefore, you must see to it on your own that your doctor is using the latest medical research as a basis for making treatment decisions. No way around it. You need to be willing to look up the guidelines and talk with your doctor about them.

Why Some Doctors Don't Use Guidelines

Reviews of doctor surveys show that the biggest barriers for doctors in using up-to-date science-based guidelines for treating patients are 1) they don't have enough information about the new guidelines, 2) they don't have enough time to learn about them, or 3) they are not ready to change their practice patterns.[5] Some doctors disagree with specific guidelines. Some feel that, especially with guidelines for counseling patients on healthy behavior, giving patients advice on how to live healthier will be useless. But as many as 20% of doctors in a number of surveys are simply stuck in their old ways of doing things and have no motivation to change.

You can see from this research that even if your doctor is one who would like to use the latest guidelines, you may need to be a full partner in the effort. Look up guidelines on your own and study the information. Bring the data you find to your doctor and be prepared to ask questions. (Be sure to ask your questions concisely and with respect for your doctor's time.) If you find that your doctor is resistant to working with you in this way, find a different doctor who either already knows the new guidelines or who is open to learning about them and who is willing to work with you to implement them.

Grace

Grace, a 59-year-old mother of six and grandmother of eleven, enjoyed a great relationship with her whole family. She also managed the electrical repair business she and her husband, Don, owned.

In February 2003, Grace began experiencing bowel problems. When the symptoms didn't go away, she went to her doctor. After running some tests, the doctor called her in and, in a somber voice, gave her the news: She had colon cancer, and he was scheduling her for surgery immediately.

Returning home still reeling from the shock of her diagnosis, Grace was assaulted by a news story about 17-year-old Jesica Santillan. The young girl had undergone a successful heart–lung transplant at the prestigious Duke University Hospital. But due to a blood-type mismatch between the organ donor and Jesica—a staff error—Jesica had died.

Shocked about her own diagnosis and scared about the surgery, Grace was horrified to think that the kind of mistake that caused Jesica's death could happen to her. How could such an awful error have been made at what was considered a very high-quality hospital, affiliated with a major university medical school? If something like that could happen there, what could happen at her small, local hospital?

Over the next couple of days, Grace read every article she could find about Jesica's case. She learned that medical errors are far more prevalent throughout the country than people realize. One article, from the National Patient Safety Foundation, said that patients could—and should—take steps to protect themselves against medical errors. This piqued her interest, so Grace went to the NPSF website.

For Grace, the NPSF website was eye-opening. She printed a news report about the Santillan case and an article that told patients how to advocate for themselves when in the hospital. She shared with her family what she had learned. Grace's son John listened intently. Because he knew Grace was hesitant about speaking up for herself, he insisted on going with her to the doctor the following day. What happened to Jesica was not going to happen to his mother—not if he had anything to say about it!

The meeting with the doctor got off to a rocky start. When Grace mentioned the materials from the website, the doctor became indignant and accused them of not trusting him. John looked him in the eye and said, "Doctor, this is my mother we're talking about here. I don't care if this offends you. I want to make sure there won't be any mistakes made with her care."

Realizing John was not about to back down, the doctor reluctantly asked to see the list of safety recommendations. As he read, he began nodding his head. By the time he had finished he agreed that John would type up his mother's medical history to keep at her hospital bedside. It would list the drugs she was taking, the drugs she was allergic to, and other information that would be useful to the medical staff.

Together they agreed that, following the NPSF recommendations, John would be with his mother much of the time she was in the hospital. Among other things, he would make sure what medications she was given while there, check the dosage amounts and frequency, and every time medication was administered he would ask what it was and the dosage level, to make sure everything was correct. He would also ask all hospital attendants if they had washed their hands before touching his mother.

With the doctor's cooperation, the plan came together quickly and easily. Then John and Grace asked the doctor detailed questions about what would be done in the surgery and what to expect afterward. With a new level of communication established between them, the doctor was very forthcoming in explaining what would be happening and what to be prepared for.

Grace went in for her surgery the next day. She wasn't thrilled to be having it, but she was much more relaxed and reassured after her meeting with the doctor. John was able to be with her much of the time over the next few days, and for the times he could not be there, other family members were. John had prepared all of them to ask the right questions and to be alert to what the hospital staff should be doing. And during the few times Grace was alone, she set aside her fears and advocated for herself, asking the questions from the patient safety guidelines.

As far as Grace and her family know, there were no medical errors in her care. Everyone, including the doctor, was well satisfied that they had all pulled together to make the experience as positive as possible. Before Grace's release from the hospital, she and John met with the doctor and asked all their questions about how to handle her care at home and afterward in chemotherapy. Now completely comfortable with the "partnership" relationship they had established, the doctor advised them in detail.

A year later, Grace's cancer was in remission, and she had returned to the full-time management of the family business. She and her family are happy that they found and used the patient safety recommendations to protect her. They had taken responsibility for Grace's health and immeasurably increased the odds of a happy outcome. It may not have been easy at times, but it was definitely worth it.

11 Medical Errors and Patient Safety

Healthcare is a decade or more behind other high-risk industries in its attention to ensuring basic safety.
—Institute of Medicine report, *To Err Is Human*, March 2000

In This Chapter...
- The widespread extent of medical errors.
- The causes of medical errors.
- Tips for preventing medical errors.

The Startling Truth About Safety

In medicine, *safety* refers to freedom from accidental injury due to a medical error. Here are some sobering statistics and unfortunate facts about the prevalence of medical errors in the United States today.

- According to the Institute of Medicine, in 2000, as many people died from medical errors as died from motor vehicle accidents (43,458), breast cancer (42,297), and AIDS (16,516) combined. Based on their 1999 landmark report, between 44,000 and 98,000 Americans die each year due to medical errors. Many thousands more suffer nonfatal injury from medical errors.[1]

- 18 key types of hospital injuries, including "foreign body left during procedure," result in 2.4 million extra days of hospitalization, $9.3 billion in excess charges, and 32,591 attributable deaths every year.[2]

- More than 770,000 people are injured or die each year in hospitals from improper drug treatment alone. These types of mistakes include giving the wrong dose size, giving the wrong drug, giving patients a drug they are known to be allergic to, giving a medication to the wrong patient, missing doses, giving duplicate doses, etc.[3]

- According to a recent *Consumer Reports* article, the odds of dying of a heart attack or in the intensive-care unit in the worst American hospitals are two times greater than in the best hospitals.[4]

- Hundreds of thousands of patients experience "near misses" of injury due to medical errors—medical mistakes where harm is narrowly escaped. Many who have these near-miss experiences never know about it because the medical staffs find little reason to inform them that they were *almost* a statistic.

- Many doctors and hospitals currently have no rigorous error-monitoring and improvement systems.

Medication errors are the most common healthcare errors.

For legal reasons, most doctors and hospitals don't disclose data about their preventable errors, even internally. This makes it difficult to study the causes of such errors. This is beginning to change, fortunately, as many hospitals and health plans try to learn from the airline industry's "blameless reporting" approach to learning from errors in order to avoid repeating them. However, many who study these problems feel improvements in patient safety are happening too slowly and blame it on providers' resistance to change.

The Keys to Avoiding Errors

Contrary to popular belief, most medical errors are not due to technical incompetence. Better training or recruiting doctors from higher-ranked medical schools isn't the big solution. Most errors result from miscommunications among the team, technical or process malfunctions, and systems glitches. Most of these are characterized as "accidents."

What does this mean? It means that *learning from past mistakes* is just as important as hiring competent staff. High-quality medical-care systems have rigorous procedures for identifying and weeding out errors (or "accidents"). It takes far more than competent staff to accomplish this. Even the most experienced medical professionals make errors, and often there are several factors involved.

The doctors and hospitals that have been shown to provide the best medical care participate in carefully organized *systems* specifically designed to monitor and enhance quality. Within these systems, studies are done to determine the exact cause of each preventable error. The lessons from each study are used to modify existing patterns of care or to improve training so as to decrease chances of the error happening again.

To provide consistently safe service, management must pay attention to all patient-care systems and processes to eliminate miscommunication, inadvertent misuse of equipment during crises, etc. Each staff member must be absolutely honest and forthright in disclosing errors so that the system can collect and analyze all relevant data.

Find out whether your medical group, hospital, and health plan can show a track record of reducing errors. You deserve to know!

Patient-to-Caregiver Communication: The Key to Your Safety

Grace's story at the start of this chapter illustrates how one woman and her family ensured her safety during her major surgery and hospital stay. Grace used recommendations from the National Patient Safety Foundation. A new program sponsored by the Joint Commission on the Accreditation of Healthcare Organizations (JCAHO) gives very similar good advice on how to better ensure your safety when getting medical care. The program, called "Speak Up," advises the following:

> The odds of dying of a heart attack or in the intensive-care unit in the worst American hospitals are two times greater than in the best hospitals.

- Speak up if you have questions or concerns, and if you don't understand, ask again. It's your body and you have the right to know.

- Pay attention to the care you are receiving. Make sure you're getting the right treatments and medications from the right healthcare professionals. Don't assume anything.

- Educate yourself about your diagnosis, the medical tests you are undergoing, and your treatment plan.

- Ask a trusted family member or friend to be your advocate.

- Know what medications you take and why you take them. Medication errors are the most common healthcare errors.

- Only use a hospital, clinic, surgery center, or other type of healthcare organization that has undergone a rigorous on-site evaluation based on established state-of-the-art quality and safety standards, such as is provided by JCAHO.

- Participate in all decisions about your treatment. You are the center of your healthcare team.

For more tips on patient safety, see *www.jcaho.org* and *www.ahrq.gov*, and check the other hospital quality websites listed in Appendix B, especially the Leapfrog Group and the National Patient Safety Foundation.

The Leapfrog Group

The Leapfrog Group is composed of more than 140 public and private organizations that provide healthcare benefits. This group identifies patient safety problems in hospitals and proposes improvements. Additionally, Leapfrog provides comparative safety information about specific hospitals as well as advice on how to avoid preventable errors for the type of care you need. See their website at *www.leapfroggroup.org* for more information.

The National Patient Safety Foundation

The National Patient Safety Foundation is a non-profit organization committed to improving the safety of patients, especially in hospitals. This organization studies causes of medical errors and provides information on best practices to hospitals and other medical care providers for improving safety. On this organization's website, *www.npsf.org*, consumers and care providers can find information about patient involvement in getting the best care and learn about improving communication between patients and their caregivers to promote safety.

> **You are the center of your healthcare team.**

If You Need to Be Hospitalized

If you have a choice, use a hospital that does a high volume of the type of care or surgery you need.

Check the Leapfrog Group website (*www.leapfrog group.org*) for data on your local hospitals and on the type of surgery you need. Also, Appendix B has other helpful information about sources of quality survey data on hospitals.

Remember, you should know about and have a say in *everything* that happens to your body while you are in a hospital. Your health should always be the focus of your care. Hospital routines should serve your needs, not the staff's or hospital's needs. Don't let yourself be intimidated by hospital staff who seem to feel otherwise. To get the best care, combine assertiveness with a partnering and empathetic approach toward staff, who may have overfull workloads.

The Agency for Healthcare Research and Quality (AHRQ) offers the following tips:

- If you are in a hospital, consider asking all healthcare workers who have direct contact with you whether they have washed their hands.

- If you are having surgery, make sure that you, your doctor, and your surgeon all agree and are clear on exactly what will be done.

- When you are being discharged from the hospital, ask your doctor to fully explain the treatment plan you will use at home.

Bad Drug Interactions

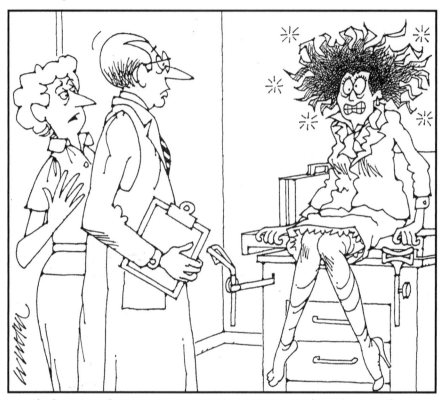

"HER TIME-RELEASE DIET PILL, TWELVE-HOUR ALLERGY CAPSULE, SEVEN-DAY DEODORANT AND ALL-DAY HAIR SPRAY ALL WENT OFF AT THE SAME TIME."

Carl

Carl is 25 and works as a programmer for a high-tech firm in the New England area. He has had asthma all his life, but has struggled with it more than ever for the last five years. Because of his illness, he misses a lot of workdays, and he has had to go to the emergency room for treatment at least twice a year for the last two years.

Carl's wife, Angela, worries about his asthma a lot. Carl's job is very stressful, often requiring him to work 12-hour days. The pay is good, though, so he has not seriously thought about finding less-stressful work. However, on one occasion after Carl went to the ER and then missed two days of work, Carl's manager told him about an employee in another department who had asthma. Apparently this other employee had switched health plans the previous year to an HMO that had a good asthma management program. The other employee had been participating in this program for several months now and had missed many fewer workdays and was in general feeling much better than before. Carl said he would like to talk with the other employee, if possible.

Carl's manager said he would ask the other employee if she would be willing to talk with Carl about her experiences. The next day, Betty, the other employee, called Carl. She told him that one of the best things about her new asthma management program was that she had been given a "peak flow meter" to use at home every day to measure the force of her exhalation. With this device, she could now tell when her asthma was getting worse and catch it before it reached crisis level. Another good thing about the program was that she had a nurse "coach" to help her make decisions about adjusting her medications according to the daily peak flow meter readings. The program had also taught her a lot about the disease and some other things she could do to help lessen its impact on her life.

Although Betty, too, had made regular trips to the ER before she started the program, she had not made one trip since. Now, she was feeling much more in control of her disease. Betty told Carl that she had felt nervous about joining an HMO, but that, in fact, her experiences had been pretty positive. She had found that the HMO provided care that was much more coordinated and comprehensive than any she had received during the years she had belonged to a PPO.

Carl, too, felt uneasy about joining an HMO. For one thing, he had been going to the same doctor for years and was uncomfortable about using a new doctor, especially an HMO doctor. When he told Angela what Betty had said, Angela also felt concerned about switching health plans. She had just seen a new gynecologist who was very nice. Angela would have to find another new gynecologist if they switched to the HMO. But this asthma management program sounded like a very good thing for Carl. Angela asked Carl to bring home all of the materials about the HMO that were provided for the company's open enrollment period, which was happening soon.

Carl brought home the HMO materials and Angela looked them over carefully. Then Angela asked a friend who was a member of this HMO about her care experiences. The friend said she had generally had very good experiences, that she liked her doctor, and that she felt she was being well cared for because her doctor made a point of keeping her up-to-date on all of the preventive tests and screenings that were important. Even when she had been very sick a couple of years ago, Angela's friend felt that her doctor did everything possible for her, including ordering extensive lab tests and authorizing surgery. Her care had cost her very little out of pocket, though she knew some of it was very expensive. Angela's friend said that, frankly, she didn't understand what all the fuss was about in the public's reaction against HMOs. At least the plan she belonged to seemed very good, and she had no complaints.

After considering what her friend had said and the advantages to Carl of the asthma management program, Angela told Carl she thought they should switch to the HMO for the next year. They should try it out, at least. If things didn't work out, they could always switch back to the PPO plan the following year.

Carl made the switch to the HMO for himself and enrolled Angela as a dependent on his plan. He found a doctor on the HMO plan that he liked and made arrangements with his new doctor to start participating in the asthma management program. He was given a peak flow meter to use daily and was put in touch with a nurse coach to help him learn to manage his disease better. Within a couple of weeks, Carl was feeling much better more of the time.

Now, several months later, Carl has yet to miss a single day of work since beginning the program, nor has he made a single trip to the ER. Angela has been able to find new doctors she likes. Both Carl and Angela are impressed with the way all of their care is much more coordinated now, compared to the care they had gotten from their old doctors and health plan. One thing that seems to make a big difference is that their care is tracked on an electronic medical record system that is used by all the doctors they see. The doctors are able to look up their medical history, prescribed medications, and lab test results on the computer very quickly. Although the next open enrollment period has not arrived yet, both Angela and Carl know that they will be staying with this health plan.

12 Coordinated Care

What we imagine is order is merely the prevailing form of chaos.
—Kerry Thornley

In This Chapter...
- U.S. healthcare is generally very unorganized.
- Better organization and coordination of care leads to better medical results.
- What you can do to get more coordinated care.

Who's Running the Show?

In a three-ring circus, many things occur at the same time. If you have been to such a circus, you know that it all seems very orderly. The high-wire act is happening in the first ring while the clowns are setting up in the second ring, and the lion tamer is just finishing up in the third ring while the juggler is waiting on the sidelines to take his place. It is very busy, but the Ring Master has everything coordinated.

One of the biggest problems with our healthcare system today is that there is no Ring Master! It is not well coordinated at all. In fact, for the most part, it is very disjointed. Experts on U.S. healthcare, such as those who served on the Institute of Medicine's Quality Committee, recognize this. But most of us don't need experts to tell us the system isn't working like it should. Unless you use a highly integrated system (see Chapter 15), you may have experienced one or more of the following situations.

- You wind up in an emergency room, and the emergency medical staff does not have access to your regular medical files.

In this situation, unless you or someone with you is able to tell the ER staff about any medication allergies, they will have no way of knowing. If you are in an auto accident, for example, and are brought in unconscious, this could be a major problem.

- Your father's cardiologist prescribes a drug that has dangerous effects when taken with a drug prescribed by a different doctor for another problem.

Without coordination, your father's health depends on either his cardiologist's remembering to inquire or your father's remembering to mention that he is taking another drug. Unfortunately, reliance upon the memory of either of the parties is statistically faulty.

- A patient has heart problems as well as osteoarthritis, and has switched orthopedic doctors three times over the last four years in search of better pain relief. The multiple specialists who treat this patient for various conditions don't communicate with each other in any way, let alone coordinate their treatment plans.

Coordination of care is critical when there is a serious or chronic health problem.

Patients who suffer from multiple chronic problems are especially vulnerable to lack of coordination. The patient's cardiologist is unlikely to be kept informed about treatments and medications prescribed by the orthopedic doctors unless either the doctor or the patient makes a special effort for this to happen, which rarely occurs. If this sharing of information does not happen, treatment and/or medications prescribed by each doctor may conflict.

What Is Coordinated Care?
The Institute of Medicine's report *Crossing the Quality Chasm* defines coordination of care as "the extent to which patient care services are coordinated across people, functions, activities, and sites over time so as to maximize the value of services delivered to patients."[1] This means delivering the necessary care to each patient when and how it is needed, even though the various elements of that care may come from different sources.

How Much Does Lack of Coordination Affect Quality?
Research shows that the better the coordination, the better the quality of the healthcare. For those of us who are in relatively good health, poor coordination of medical resources is just an irritation that may not present any real adverse effects. For example, if you're basically well but have trouble getting your records transferred to a new doctor when you move or switch health plans, you probably won't suffer any adverse health effects. However, if you are seriously ill, having your records transferred quickly can be important. Likewise, if you are basically well, having your specialist and primary-

care doctors communicate with each other is good but not crucial, whereas this communication is more life-impacting the more ill you are.

Coordination of care is critical when there is a serious or chronic health problem. Poorly coordinated care is especially risky when a patient has multiple and simultaneous chronic health problems. For example, consider the situation of an older person who has serious complications of diabetes while he is receiving chemotherapy for colon cancer. Medication or treatment given for one of these problems could interfere with that given for the other.

> Patients who suffer from multiple chronic problems are especially vulnerable to lack of coordination.

Medical Families Face Challenges Too

Even doctors have difficulty finding high-quality medical care, especially well-coordinated care, for their family members. For example, the Agency for Healthcare Research and Quality recently reported the following: Even patients who have a knowledgeable physician in the family to act as their advocate face challenges in receiving good medical care, concludes Frederick M. Chen, MD, M.P.H., of the Agency for Healthcare Research and Quality.

Dr. Chen and his colleagues invited chairpersons of U.S. academic departments of family medicine to describe recent experiences with the healthcare system when a parent of theirs was seriously ill. In-depth interviews were conducted with eight family physicians who had been practicing for an average of 19 years and who wanted to talk about their parent's healthcare experiences.

These doctors witnessed numerous obstacles to quality care, such as poor communication and fragmented care, which in many cases compelled them to intervene—to "rescue" their parent from medical mistakes. They were concerned about their parent's care and felt that the system did not work the way it should. They suggested that patients might receive better treatment if healthcare systems reinforced the role of an accountable attending physician, encouraged continuity of care, and emphasized knowing the patient as a person.

The informed views of these doctors raise serious concerns about how well the healthcare system is serving patients.[2]

Case Management

If you become seriously ill, you will most likely need care from multiple providers. If you suffer a stroke, for example, you will need a primary-care physician as well as a neurologist. You may also require a physical therapist, someone to monitor your blood-thinning medication, and perhaps a speech therapist, plus someone to advise you and your family how to modify your home.

Good medical care systems have "case management" programs that coordinate care among all the appropriate types of providers for each seriously ill patient. Case management means that medical resources are coordinated so as to ensure that all prescribed care is given in a timely way. In good case management programs, each seriously ill patient is assigned a staff liaison—usually a nurse—called a "case manager." A good case manager not only makes sure all of the patient's care is well coordinated, but also monitors the patient's progress, letting providers know when prescribed care isn't working as planned and alerting them to the need to modify the care.

Good case management thus promotes high quality as well as cost-effectiveness. It ensures that the patient receives all needed care but no unnecessary care. A number of health plans and insurance companies provide case management services for their highest-cost patients. Many are making case management a key component of their chronic disease management programs.

Disease Management

Good healthcare systems have also implemented "disease management processes." The story about Carl at the beginning of this chapter is about a disease management program for asthma. It is an illustration of what a disease management program can do to improve health. Various types of these programs are available from some health plans and some doctors and doctor groups. If you have a chronic disease, you should investigate which of the doctors and health plans available to you offer a disease management program that could help you with your illness. The most common types of these programs are for diabetes, heart disease, and asthma.

Disease management is different from case management in the following way: Very seriously ill patients receive case management. This includes people with multiple chronic and/or acute medical problems who need their care coordinated. Disease management processes, by contrast, are designed around

> Good medical care systems have "case management" programs that coordinate care among all the appropriate types of providers for each seriously ill patient.

specific chronic diseases, like diabetes. All patients who have diabetes at any stage of the illness, whether mild or severe, could be included in a diabetes management program. If a patient has both diabetes and asthma, he or she could be included in two disease management programs, one for diabetes and one for asthma. Some plans even have disease management programs able to address "co-morbidities"—the medical term for having multiple conditions—at the same time.

By targeting patients who have specific common conditions, creating large-scale patient education and assistance programs focusing on each disease, and providing information to doctors about the treatments that have been proven to work best for each of these diseases, disease management has led to healthier, more satisfied patients and to more motivated and prepared providers.

A Disease Management Model
Disease management includes both the coordination of care and additional services to assist in the management of a chronic illness. For example, the best disease management programs often include an assigned nurse case manager who stays in touch with you and teaches you how to treat your illness at home. In the very best health plans, outreach programs—in which nurses call members at home—include not only chronic disease patients but also patients at risk of developing chronic diseases, women with at-risk pregnancies, as well as others who can benefit from getting information about their medical conditions, help in managing their conditions, and reminders for needed preventive care services.

Conditions most often targeted for disease management programs are heart disease, heart failure, asthma, diabetes, and depression. Other conditions targeted include those where treatment costs and prevalence are high, where there is good scientific evidence about treatments that work best, where there is high variation in the treatments doctors prescribe, and where services to patients are fragmented. Good disease management programs address all of these problems effectively.

Elements of good disease management are:
- Teams of providers working closely together, maximizing the unique skills of each team participant, and providing the full set of expertise needed by each patient.

- Good collection of outcome measurement information (how well a patient is doing at each step of care) and feedback of this information to all team providers.

> The larger the medical group, the more likely it will have the financial and other resources needed to implement good disease management programs.

- Use of scientific evidence that shows providers the best treatments for the condition.

- Patient education and support about how best to participate as a member on his or her own healthcare team.

- Use of computer-aided support tools.

Can You Get Good Disease Management?

Research shows that your chances of getting the best disease management for a chronic illness are less than 50/50. Four chronic diseases affect almost half of all people with a chronic illness: congestive heart failure, diabetes, asthma, and depression. Researchers at the University of California surveyed 1,040 medical groups and independent physician practice associations across the U.S. to determine if the best practices for disease management of these four chronic illnesses were being used.

Don't assume coordination exists unless your provider explicitly tells you it does.

On average, the surveyed physician groups use only 5 of 16 recommended disease management processes. No physician group surveyed had implemented all recommended disease management processes for all four diseases. Only groups with at least 20 participating physicians were surveyed because smaller groups are even less likely to have the resources to implement the recommended management processes.[3]

About 125 million of the 276 million people in the U.S. have a chronic illness. If half of these have one of the four most common illnesses, then the other half have less common illnesses for which good disease management is even less prevalent. Also, even if they have one of the four most common chronic diseases, many people receive their care from a doctor who does not belong to a medical group with 20 or more physicians and who therefore is unlikely to have the resources to implement the best disease management. What this boils down to is that your chances of getting the best medical management for a chronic illness are mighty slim.

The larger the medical group, the more likely it will have the financial and other resources needed to implement good disease management programs. This makes sense. The above-mentioned survey also found that better information technology is high on the list of resources that can best assist physicians in implementing these programs. Additionally, the survey found that the physician groups implementing the best disease management programs tend to be motivated by getting better health plan contracts or higher pay for providing better-quality care.

Two Secrets to Getting Better Coordinated Care

There is not much you can do to improve coordination of the entire U.S. healthcare system, but you can know what options are available to you. Here are two suggestions.

Be Inquisitive

Don't assume coordination exists unless your provider explicitly tells you it does. The time to look into such matters is before, not after, an unfortunate and avoidable error occurs. Ask your providers direct questions such as:

- "How thoroughly and how often do you share information about my care with my other providers?"

- "Am I in a system, for example, where the medications to which I am allergic are known by all of my providers through computer tracking?"

  If not, you may want to take some precautions of your own, such as attaching a note to your driver's license about your allergies. Make sure to notify all of your doctors and other care providers about your allergies to medications. It would be a good idea to create a written document listing your major health problems, medications, and allergies. Make sure your family members and/or friends know where it is in case they need to give it to healthcare providers treating you.

- "Is the care I am getting from you communicated to the specialists treating my other medical problems?"

  If not, you need to ask your specialists to communicate with one another as well as with your primary-care doctor thoroughly and appropriately to make sure your care is well coordinated.

- "Are the results of my lab tests available to all my doctors— without my actually taking the results to each of them?"

  If not, take or send copies of the results to all your doctors.

Take Charge of Your Own Well-Being

You must be willing to take on the role of coordinating your own (or a family member's) care. If it is not being done by your medical-care sources, you must play the role. You may need to create your own tracking systems to monitor and report all aspects of care, including multiple drugs taken and changes in health status.

In this role, you may need to become expert at accessing information about available resources, including free or low-

> You must be willing to take on the role of coordinating your own or a family member's care.

cost programs in your community. You may want to tap into the vast amount of information on the Internet about specific diseases and their management. See Appendix A for information on trustworthy Internet sources of medical information.

Sandy

This is the story of a woman whose health crisis was amplified by having to search for a doctor at the last minute. She did not have time to find a doctor she could be sure offered high-quality care or with whom she felt comfortable working. Unfortunately, the physician she ended up with had a gruff, off-putting manner that made her feel awkward about asking questions and discussing controversial issues. This patient survived her crisis but it wasn't without tough times.

Sandy is a 45-year-old mother of two daughters, one just out of college and one still in college. Sandy has been working professionally for the last 15 years. Three years ago she left her employer of 12 years to take a higher-level position with another firm. Her new company did not offer the group-model HMO she had belonged to for 12 years, so Sandy joined the company's PPO health plan. Her new plan did not require her to choose a primary-care physician when she signed up. Because she was extremely busy in her new position, she did not take the time to look for a new primary-care doctor.

A year later, Sandy realized she should get her annual well-woman exam. She looked at her plan's list of doctors and called several of them. One doctor she called was not accepting new patients, another could not see her for four months, and the last one was no longer a member of the health plan. Sandy had hoped to get an appointment before her next busy work season, which was coming up fast, so she vowed to keep looking for a doctor on the list who could see her soon. However, she got involved in a new project and did not call any more doctors.

One day at work, Sandy tripped and fell softly against the hallway wall. She was not injured, but she felt a sharp pain in her right breast. At home that night, she discovered a lump she had never noticed before. In a panic, she called her health plan and explained that she needed to find a doctor on the plan's list immediately.

Sandy's plan's customer service representative gave her the phone numbers for half a dozen doctors in her area. She called each one on the list until she found one who could see her immediately. After a very short appointment the next day, the doctor sent Sandy across the street to the hospital for a mammogram. That same afternoon, the doctor called her to schedule a biopsy to remove the lump, which was done two days later. The lab results confirmed Sandy had a malignancy.

The doctor mentioned briefly that there were some alternative treatments but said tersely that he strongly recommended the full removal of her entire breast and other related tissue. Sandy asked the doctor some questions, which he answered with short sentences. The doctor pressed Sandy to set a date for surgery, and though she felt very uneasy about not exploring her options, she felt pressured to comply with the doctor's recommendation.

Sandy set a date for surgery, then instantly burst into tears, feeling lost, out-of-control, and panicked about her future. She wasn't comfortable with her new doctor but did not feel she had time to find another one. For one thing, she lacked the energy to search for a new doctor, having to put all her energy into dealing with her very serious illness.

Two years later, after a mastectomy and months of radiation therapy, Sandy's cancer seemed to be in remission. At this point she was thoroughly fed up with her physician and was determined to find a new one. Even though he had gotten her through the breast cancer alive, for which she was grateful, she had experienced many problems in her recovery. The doctor continued to treat her in a way she felt was disrespectful and arrogant.

The human resources (HR) manager for her company told Sandy about a quality survey of many physician groups in her state, including local groups, that had been sponsored and publicized by the state government. The HR manager told Sandy where to find the information on the Internet and explained that she might want to find a doctor who was part of one of the more highly rated medical groups. She recommended using the website of the medical group of her choice and calling its customer service number for assistance in finding doctors who were taking new patients and whom she could interview. Sandy did exactly that, and she paid the co-payments for two office visits to meet with two doctors. She chose one, has been seeing that doctor for the past year, and is very happy with her choice. Fortunately, her breast cancer remains in remission.

Sandy has also read up on all the other types of preventive care she should be getting. She regularly shares with her doctor the preventive and other medical guidelines she finds on good Internet cites and discusses with him the treatments that may apply to her situation as well as what can be learned from the latest medical research. Sandy now has peace of mind knowing that she has a physician who works as her partner. Though the effects of this peace of mind and partnership can't be measured, they undoubtedly will improve her health.

Sandy strongly regrets that she did not go through a more careful doctor search process before she had her breast cancer crisis. She urges friends and colleagues to find a good doctor who will work with them *before* they have some medical crisis.

13 Patient-Centered Care

The dedicated physician is constantly striving for a balance between personal, human values, scientific realities, and the inevitabilities of God's will.

—Dr. David Allman

In This Chapter...
- Healthcare is not very customer-focused.
- Currently, most healthcare is set up more for the convenience of providers than for that of consumers.
- Care that is convenient to use leads to patients getting better care.
- The medical care system doesn't always respect patients as full human beings.
- Medical care needs to fully recognize that our humanity comes with many variations.
- You should insist on being treated with respect and dignity.

The Patient As Customer

Sandy's story on the preceding pages shows how care can be distinctly improved from the patient's perspective when mutual respect and true partnership are at the heart of the doctor–patient relationship.

The business community learned long ago that the way to gain greater market share is to provide superior service. For example, in the mid-1980s Nordstrom department store made headlines with its pioneering work as a customer-focused retailer. Nordstrom's management took "the customer is always right" to new levels, and the store's reputation soared as it rode the wave of popularity for many years.

In a monopoly—like a utility company or a city government—there is little incentive for improving service or quality. However, non-monopolistic enterprises compete for customer loyalty. Quality and service are often primary reasons customers buy from a particular company. Convenience is an-

Patients Treated with Respect?

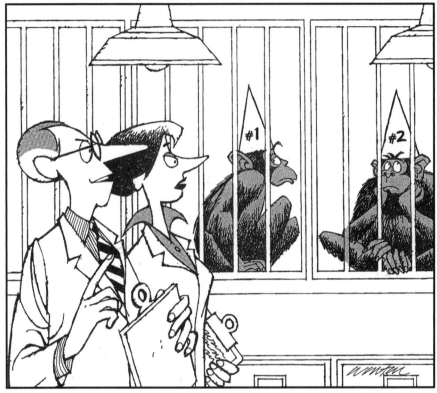

"I'VE FINALLY GOT THOSE UNRULY
PATIENTS UNDER CONTROL."

other attraction. Innovative industries come up with efficient ways to meet the needs and desires of their customers.

Imagine a world where patients were actually treated as valued customers. Imagine health plans that were designed for *your* convenience, not that of the doctors and administrators. Imagine plans that continued to offer more and more benefits for less and less money while simultaneously increasing the quality of the care you receive.

This is how most businesses operate. Look at the technology industry! As more and more manufacturers compete for our business, prices plummet, dependability increases, and warranties expand. Following are some thoughts about customer-focused healthcare.

Whose Convenience Counts?

Most healthcare today is set up to be convenient for providers and administrators. Consumers' needs are considered after those of the doctors and health plans. This approach is a remnant from times past, when the doctor was considered more important than the patient. In business, they'd say the system is not very "customer-focused."

In fact, we take this arrangement so much for granted that both consumers and healthcare industry insiders who read this may think I am making too much of an unimportant issue. But the issue is very important.

Why? Because some patients who need care avoid or delay getting it because it is too inconvenient. In systems where care is structured for the convenience of the providers, plan managers, and administrators, patients are not encouraged to establish strong, mutually responsible, and mutually respectful partnerships with providers.

Here are some points to consider:

- **Daytime hours:** Most doctor appointments are available only during the workday. Therefore, if we need a doctor's help, many of us have to take time off from our own jobs to get it. Sometimes this is very difficult. Having some evening and/or weekend appointments available would help.

- **Making appointments:** To make an appointment for a doctor's office visit, we usually must make a call during our own work hours, often spending long periods of time "on hold" or waiting for a call back. This is merely inconvenient for most people, but can be a roadblock for those whose only daytime phone access for personal calls is during a short work break. For people with Internet access, making appointments online would be much more convenient. For others, being able to set an appointment quickly and efficiently with someone by phone would be very helpful. Having this ability outside of the 8-5 time slot would make appointment-setting much easier.

- **Lack of privacy:** Discussing one's medical problems from work can be awkward, especially for people who sit in office cubicles with very little privacy. Here again, for those with Internet access, being able to communicate with a doctor or his or her staff online would resolve this problem. For others, a solution would be having phone access to physicians or their office staff, as appropriate, outside of the 8-5 time slot.

- **Unnecessary office visits:** Many doctors are paid only for office visits, not for giving medical advice to their patients by phone. As a result, they may require in-person appointments even when an office visit isn't really necessary. Health plans could devise ways to reimburse physicians for phone and email consultations. (See Chapter 16 for more on communicating by email with doctors.)

- **Waiting:** Once we actually get to the doctor's office for an appointment, we often face long delays. As patients we are expected to take extra time out of our day to accommodate the doctor's delay. Granted, the delay may be due to someone else's medical emergency, but greater respect for patients' time could make this kind of situation less frequent.

- **Specialist access:** If we must first see our primary-care physician in order to be referred to a specialist, it can take months and at least two half-days of missed work just to get a problem diagnosed. This can involve a time commitment of up to several hours for the patient and only a few minutes for the physicians. Referrals to specialists could be done much more smoothly, quickly, and with more respect for the patient's time.

For example, as in a few current systems, specialists who work in the same locations as primary-care physicians could leave time in their schedules to be called into the primary-care physician's office whenever a patient problem needed a quick specialist assessment. This eliminates a second appointment entirely. It also makes it possible to start appropriate treatment more quickly and thereby creates a better chance of solving or slowing the problem before it gets worse.

- **Finding physicians:** Relocating to a new city or changing health plans often requires making new medical-care connections. Increasingly, we also find ourselves seeking new doctors when our doctors drop out of our health plan's network. The system does not make these transitions easy. Obtaining information about doctors in our new community or our new health plan and getting set up as a patient with a new doctor can be expensive and time-consuming, requiring possibly unnecessary office visits.

Again, the costs in time and effort often cause us to wait until we are in dire need of attention before we make new connections. Better online data comparing the quality of all physicians and medical groups in all geographic areas of the country would be of enormous use to consumers. Easier ways to make connections with new physicians would also be extremely helpful.

No current healthcare systems incorporate all of these desired features and technological tools. However, some convenience and efficiency services are now offered by some systems. All improvements to convenience for consumers improve healthcare. Remember, we as consumers can speak up about what we want, and we can have influence by choosing providers who offer convenient services.

> Most healthcare today is set up to be convenient for providers and administrators. Consumers' needs are considered after those of the doctors and health plans.

Are We Really Just Body Parts?

Our nation's healthcare system has a long history of doctors dealing with patients as collections of body parts. This is a by-product of the industrialization of society that's occurred over the past few centuries, which coincided with a huge emphasis on mechanistic science. Thus, medical care has become incredibly specialized—divided into internal medicine, obstetrics and gynecology, cardiology, and a whole gaggle of other "ologies." From this perspective, a patient's humanity is sometimes seen as superfluous—interfering with the care process.

Many healthcare providers seem to be annoyed at having to deal with each of us as full-fledged human beings with distinct personalities. It is so much easier to deal with us as if we were robots! Psychologists call this "objectification"—seeing another person as an object or an "it."

Referring to people by labels further enables this phenomenon, such as when we identify people by their roles. Politicians see their constituents as "voters." Postal workers can see people as "addressees." Some healthcare professionals see their customers as "patients." Objectification makes the other person a thing. Our rationale then tells us we don't need an emotional connection as we would with a fellow human being.

Objectification sometimes makes a job more bearable; bomber pilots and artillery officers will tell you this in times of war. Some doctors may objectify patients to make their work more tolerable, especially if they specialize in an area of medical care like oncology (cancer treatment), in which they simply can't save many of their patients.

Besides being hierarchical or dismissive, objectifying people is also disrespectful. This is why women get so angry when they are seen merely as "sex objects" by men. Treating people as real human beings requires an emotional investment and a willingness to connect with the other person.

> Remember, you are the customer, and the system should be designed to serve you.

Respecting Individuality

Not only are people human beings first and customers second, each one of us is quite different. The United States is home to a uniquely diverse population, and all industries dealing with the American public must take this into account. Unique cultural differences make for highly varied responses to marketing, delivery, communication, and use of products and services.

Because health issues can trigger strong emotions in people, medical caregivers are likely to encounter an even wider range of customer personalities and preferences. A healthcare facility that strives to deliver quality must pay attention to the following types of patient differences, as well as many others:

- Ethnicity, culture, and primary language
- Religious beliefs and philosophies
- Mental capacity to comprehend medical information
- Personality and attitude
- Expectations
- Level of fear or confusion about their condition
- Level of concern about their ability to pay
- Willingness to actively participate in and take responsibility for their health.

The "Respect Gap"

When there is a "respect gap," the customer can sense it—even when the provider has a pleasant "bedside manner." Respectful service is not only a good business practice for providers for attracting and retaining customers, it is also effective in delivering high-quality medical care.

Here are a few negative effects when respect is absent in healthcare:

- **Quality diminishes:** As consumers, we can usually sense, if only on an unconscious level, when providers view us as merely "cases." When medical personnel ignore or discount important aspects of who we are, or when they treat us with overt disrespect, we feel less connected with the system that provides our care. We are less willing to engage with them, which ultimately affects our health.

- **Effectiveness decreases:** There is a small but growing recognition among care providers that treatments produce better results when they are administered with attention to the individual's unique circumstances and concerns. Treatments are more effective when the person being treated fully engages in the process—proactively choosing the treatment on the basis of being informed. Treatment must be based on mutual respect between the patient and each member of the healthcare team. On the other hand, when this doesn't happen, effectiveness of treatment decreases.

- **The "gap" widens:** When the respect gap is allowed to persist, the myth that the doctor is somehow better than the customer—his or her time is more valuable or he or she is more important as a person—is perpetuated. In turn, the public's cynicism and resignation about the state of our healthcare system grows. A resigned and cynical public does not make for a healthy healthcare system!

Demand Respect

Despite the widespread hopelessness that permeates the psyche of almost everyone associated with the healthcare system in this country—providers, plan administrators, and consumers alike—the system can be changed.

So what can you and I do? At an absolute minimum, we must demand courteous interactions from everyone in the healthcare system. This requires us to provide instant feedback when we encounter rudeness, to report any unskillful treatments, to stand willing to "fire" anyone who isn't treating us respectfully and skillfully, and to feel solid in our esteem as customers who have every right to insist upon competent and courteous healthcare.

We can influence the prevailing industry indifference by taking more ownership of our care and treatment. As long as providers have total control over medical care decisions, many doctors and other healthcare personnel will cling to the perception that courtesy and respect are nice but not essential features of the care process. When we take more control of and responsibility for our healthcare, we are far less likely to be treated as a collection of body parts. We command respect as partners in maintaining good health.

In a healthcare system dedicated to high-quality care and customer-centered service, providers will find impersonal care to be unacceptable and will exhibit an uncompromising attitude of respect for each individual. To be effective, personal service will need to permeate every level of the organization. Starting with front-line clerks, employees involved with any aspect of healthcare would be hired for their compassion and courtesy as well as for other talents and skills. Training and ongoing performance evaluations would reinforce this emphasis on patient-oriented service.

Remember, you are the customer, and the system should be designed to serve you.

CAHPS: A Resource for Evaluating Respect

As mentioned previously, in the early 1990s, leaders in healthcare quality recognized the need to obtain evaluations from the people who have received care. The idea was that, although methods existed for determining how well providers were technically providing care, a way was needed to measure how well providers were doing in the areas of communication with patients, timeliness of providing service, responsiveness, and ease of access to care. The creation of the Consumer Assessment of Health Plans Survey (CAHPS) was coordinated by the Agency for Healthcare Research and Quality (AHRQ) to answer this need. This survey also assesses clinical quality in ways not easily accessible via other means, e.g., counseling for smoking cessation.

Thousands of Americans have completed the survey, and more than 90 million Americans can get information on the plans they are offered by looking at the CAHPS results. See Appendix B under the reference for AHRQ for website information on where to get CAHPS results. Remember, though, that CAHPS measures patient satisfaction with non-clinical aspects of care. To get a combination of clinical and non-clinical aspects of care, look at a combination of surveys, such as CAHPS and HEDIS, both available at *www.ncqa.org.*

Edgar

Edgar lives in a small midwestern community. Like many men, he does not like to go to doctors. However, last year when he started feeling a tightness in his chest he got worried about having a heart attack. Edgar decided to see a local family doctor recommended by a friend. When he went to the appointment, an echocardiogram was performed in the doctor's office for Edgar. The doctor sent the test results to the cardiologist he referred Edgar to. When Edgar went to the appointment with the cardiologist, the doctor said he could not use the echocardiogram done by the family doctor. So Edgar had a second echocardiogram done in the specialist's office. When Edgar got the Explanation of Benefits statement from his insurance company, it turned out that the insurance was not going to pay for the second test, so Edgar would have to pay the full cost of that echocardiogram, which was expensive. Edgar was pretty angry about this. He had no control over what his doctors recommended. The insurance company seemed to be saying that Edgar should somehow have avoided having the second test done. It did not seem reasonable that he should be expected to take a risk with his health by telling the cardiologist not to redo the test.

After having an angry conversation with a customer service representative of the insurance company on the phone, Edgar sent a complaint letter to the insurance company about the claim denial. The insurance company wrote back to Edgar saying they would reverse their decision and would pay the claim since Edgar had no control over the care he had received. They explained that they had investigated the situation with the following results: The first echocardiogram should not have been done by the family doctor because echocardiograms are very specialized tests that require special training even for cardiologists. The cardiologist was right to repeat the test because it had been done poorly the first time. As the result of Edgar's situation and several other similar cases where echocardiograms had been inappropriately done by family doctors in the local community, the insurance company had notified all of the community doctors that it would no longer pay for echocardiograms performed in family physicians' offices.

Managed Care

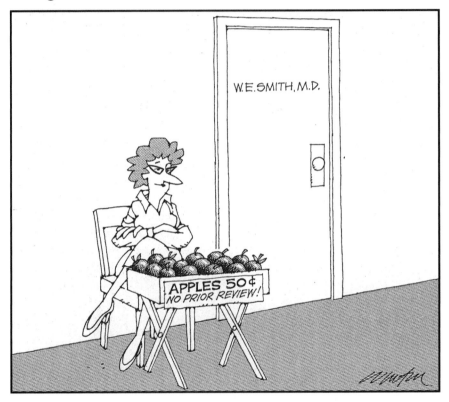

14 Managed Care

*I am neither especially clever nor especially gifted.
I am only very, very curious.* —Albert Einstein

What Is Managed Care?

The term *managed care* is confusing to most consumers. Many believe it is interchangeable with *HMO care*, which they often associate with poor quality. Actually, managed care is any activity that is set up to control either costs or quality or both—in *all* types of plans, not just HMOs.

Insurance companies and health plans developed managed care processes to curb the free spending and runaway cost increases that accompany the uncontrolled fee-for-service practice of medicine. Under fee-for-service, opportunistic providers can give unnecessary treatments so they can invoice for the services—sometimes without regard to the increased health risk to the patient. This practice becomes even more widespread when the full tab is picked up by the insurance company or by Medicare.

At its best, managed care yields the highest-quality care, because it builds in mechanisms to ensure that patients receive only the most effective care in the most effective way at the most appropriate time. This is also the best way to keep costs under control. When costs are reduced by skimping on needed care or by cutting corners on quality, patients can get sicker and then require even more care than they would have needed if all the right care had been given initially.

Unfortunately, some plans use managed care rules solely to control costs and not to ensure quality. The objective for these plans isn't higher quality—just increased profits. However, many plans use managed care *both* to improve quality *and* to control costs—an appropriate approach, as long as quality is the primary goal.

Who's Doing the Managing?

For the most part, the managing in "managed care" is done directly by health plans and insurance companies. The health plan determines the managed care rules and procedures it wants to use, then lists these rules in the contracts with all physicians, hospitals, and other providers who agree to be on the health plan's "in-network" list. All contracting providers agree to abide by the rules in the contract. Sometimes the health plan or insurance company subcontracts with another company, called a "utilization review" organization, which is given authority to implement managed care rules.

Rules to Expect With Managed Care

Edgar's story at the beginning of this chapter is an example of how managed care rules developed by insurance companies benefit patients (providing the most effective care in the most efficient way) while keeping costs lower (eliminating unnecessary costs). In cases where tests are invasive, such as amniocentesis, not authorizing unnecessary tests can prevent harm to the patient from possible side effects, thus also avoiding the extra costs of care for the side effects.

The following are some examples of managed care rules:

- *Requiring preauthorization by the health plan (or the utilization review company) for all elective surgeries.* Many surgeries may not be necessary. Sometimes a less-invasive and equally effective treatment exists. Requiring the physician to justify the necessity of each elective surgery is a good way to both eliminate unnecessary expenses and make sure the patient is not exposed to undue risk.

- *Requiring preauthorization for many types of out-of-network care.* Many insurance companies offer PPOs and other types of health plans that allow members to use noncontracted (out-of-network) providers. These providers have no incentive to contain costs of care. Also, the insurance company has no control over the level of quality of these providers. To maintain some degree of cost and quality control, many insurance companies require that certain types of care from noncontracted providers get their approval before they will pay anything toward that care.

- *Having "formulary" lists of approved drugs.* Most insurance companies negotiate with multiple drug manufacturers for the best volume purchasing deals they can get. If they can get a better price for one drug that is claimed to be equivalent to another more costly drug, they put the less-expensive drug on their "formulary" list. Each plan creates its own formulary list, so the lists tend to be somewhat (but not hugely) different from plan to plan.

The more often insurance companies can induce you to use these less-costly drugs, the less prescription drug coverage costs. Lower copayments motivate patients to request formulary-listed drugs from their doctors. If an insurance company makes sure that drugs on its formulary are good substitutes for those not on the formulary, then it is doing a good job of "managed care" in relation to its drug coverage.

Choosing a highly rated HMO may be your best, easiest way to get high-quality care.

- *Requiring primary-care physicians to refer to specialists.* Twenty years ago, many HMOs contracted with primary-care physicians in such a way that the physician lost money when referring a patient to a specialist. The primary physician had to give up part of his or her payment from the HMO to pay the specialist. This discouraged some specialist referrals, even when they were clinically appropriate.

This type of contracting is for the most part no longer done. Primary-care physicians in most HMOs no longer have a financial incentive to avoid referring patients to specialists. However, specialist care can be expensive. Therefore most HMO plans want to make sure members need specialist care before they are willing to pay for it. This is one reason HMOs usually require your primary physician to refer you to a specialist if you need to see one. The primary physician no longer has to pay for the referral; he or she only has to make sure you need to see the specialist. Another reason for this rule is that patients get the best results when care is well coordinated. The primary-care physician is in the best position to orchestrate this coordination.

Is managed care "bad" for consumers? Only when it is used to control costs at the expense of quality. How can you tell if this is happening? Use quality-of-care surveys to see which plans are achieving the highest ratings. See Appendix B for sources of these reports.

If you choose another type of plan over an HMO because you want to avoid managed care, you may not get the best value for your dollar unless you are willing to become very knowledgeable and assertive about getting what you need and coordinating your care. Choosing a highly rated HMO may be your best, easiest way to get high-quality care.

Fears About Managed Care

Consumers' main fear about managed care is that they will be denied care they really need. If you share this fear, the following may reassure you. According to a *Journal of the American Medical Association* study, nearly 60% of member appeals to two large California HMOs did not involve any question about the medical necessity of a procedure. Fifty-seven percent of all appeals were requesting coverage for gastric bypass surgery (stomach stapling), breast alteration surgery, or varicose vein removal. These are all procedures that have to be considered very carefully on a case-by-case basis to determine their appropriateness and necessity. You might also like to know that during the appeals process, the HMOs decided 41.9% of all appeals in favor of the member, overturning some of the plan's original decisions.[1]

Handling Disagreements

If you disagree with your managed care plan's proposed treatment, follow these steps to ensure you get the care you deserve.

1. Work with your doctor to sort out what the latest scientific research shows to be the best treatment for your diagnosis.

2. Do your own research using trustworthy sources to find out what evidence-based guidelines have been established for treating your condition.

3. If you and your doctor agree that you should have a certain type of care that your plan is denying you, appeal the decision. If you can show valid evidence in support of the requested treatment, your chances are good of having the denial reversed.

4. If you still disagree with the health plan's final decision about your care, seek out state-level resources that can help you determine the legitimacy of your claim against your HMO. (If your plan is a PPO or other non-HMO type, government-level assistance may be limited, but check what is available to you.)

When costs are reduced by skimping on needed care or by cutting corners on quality, patients can get sicker and then require even more care than they would have needed if all the right care had been given initially.

Here's an example. In California, an independent review board of medical experts is available through the State Department of Managed Care to review grievances about HMOs. The board has decided in favor of consumers in approximately half of its cases, using the latest in scientific research as its guide. This indicates that the consumers whose cases are not supported by this board may not be getting sound medical advice when advised to challenge their health plan's decisions. However, if a consumer believes the health plan's decision does not offer the best treatment, it is worth the effort to bring the case to the independent review board.

Tony

Tony is a tall man, 62 years old, with very distinguished gray hair and a kind of craggy handsomeness. He'd been experiencing some odd and disturbing symptoms recently. He decided to see his doctor, who told him he needed to have certain tests to confirm whether or not he had thyroid disease. Tony felt somewhat panicked by the possibility of having this medical problem. His doctor said to make an appointment with him to discuss the results 10 days after having the tests done, so that the doctor could be sure to have the results at the appointment. Then, if the diagnosis was confirmed, his doctor would refer him to an appropriate specialist.

When Tony tried to make an appointment at the lab, he was told the first available appointment was not for another week. Therefore, Tony would have to wait two-and-a-half weeks to find out whether or not his thyroid was malfunctioning. Then it might be even a few more weeks before he could see the specialist, if necessary, to get started on treatment. This was very frustrating; Tony did not know how he would be able to make it through the next couple of weeks without knowing his health status.

Tony had met a doctor the previous weekend at his grandson's birthday party who worked for a clinic-based integrated system of care. In discussing medical care with this doctor, she had mentioned some impressive third-party-validated statistics about the high level of quality of the care given by her organization. Tony decided to contact this doctor to see if she had any suggestions. When she called him back, she said she was very sorry that Tony was not a member of the health plan whose members she treated. She said that if Tony had seen a doctor in her system, the doctor would have been able to make arrangements with the in-house lab to have the thyroid function tests done that same day, with the results returned to the doctor within 24 hours. If tests confirmed the tentative diagnosis, the doctor would be able to call in a specialist to see Tony the day she got the test results. And in fact, her system had a special treatment program already set up for people with that diagnosis. Tony would begin treatment, if necessary, within 48 hours of originally seeing her, and she would coordinate with the specialist to make sure the ongoing treatment was effective. She explained that it was the integration of all services and medical care within their system that made all this possible.

Since there was no way Tony could at that point become a member of the health plan that gave access to her system, the integrated system doctor could only confirm for Tony that the test authorized by his doctor was one of the tests he needed. She also recommended that Tony have two other tests, which she would have ordered had Tony been her patient. She suggested that Tony call his doctor and ask if he would prescribe these additional tests.

Tony was very frustrated, but there was nothing he could do except talk with his doctor about getting the additional tests, keep trying to get in sooner to have the tests done, and push hard to get a timely appointment with the specialist if it became necessary.

15 Integrated Care Systems

Failure is the opportunity to begin again more intelligently.
—Henry Ford

In This Chapter...
- What is "integration" in healthcare?
- Why integration is important.
- Very little U.S. medical care is integrated.
- Prospects for the future.

Today's very best medical care comes from comprehensive healthcare organizations called "integrated systems"—a term that means a system that pulls together all parts of the puzzle to maximize customers' health. The approach is based on a "whole-system" perspective. Tony's story shows one patient's view of the value of integrated systems of care over the disjointed and uncoordinated nature of care outside of these systems. Unfortunately, most of U.S. medical care is not integrated.

The concept of integration is confusing, even for many providers. That's one reason there is so little true integration in the industry. Let me try to make it as clear as possible.

Integrated vs. Coordinated Care

Integrated and coordinated care share the same goal: to make the delivery of your healthcare services seamless to you. The difference is that care can be coordinated by anyone (including you) who is willing to organize and track it, and to make sure you get exactly what you need and no more. In contrast, integration refers specifically to providers of all types cooperating to accomplish this goal through pre-established processes. In an integrated system, the linked providers stand ready to serve you in a coordinated way, including some ways that you may not need right now but could need at a later time.

The Healthcare Team Concept

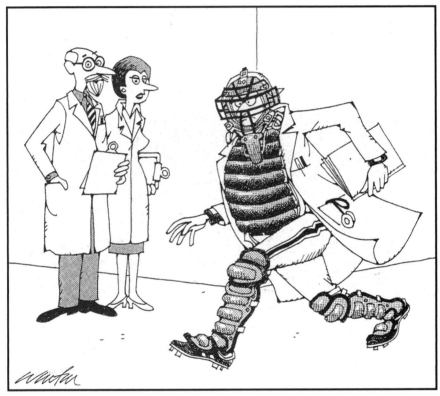

"I THINK GEORGE IS TAKING THIS
HEALTHCARE TEAM IDEA TOO FAR."

The type of integration that can make your healthcare seamless is known as "vertical integration."[1] In vertical integration of healthcare services, all types of providers and services are linked and coordinated. This is not the same as the horizontal integration that occurs when separate hospitals merge into one hospital system. Horizontal integration benefits the hospitals themselves, decreasing administrative costs and increasing bargaining power with health plans. Bringing multiple hospitals together does not help make complete care seamless for consumers, except perhaps in some minor ways.

Vertical integration links physicians, hospitals, and all other providers of care to make it easier for patients to get the care they need. One example of how this works is when a hospital or hospital system shares your medical records with your doctors, so there are not multiple sets of your records. Another example of vertical integration is when your prescription drug coverage coordinates directly with your doctor so that you do not have to act as the go-between, linking the two.

Integration does not necessarily mean that all parts of the system are under common ownership. It does, however, mean a common commitment, through both legal contracts and the attitudes of all participants, to enhancing the overall quality and seamlessness of care received by the consumer.

Integrated vs. Managed Care

How does integration differ from managed care? First, let me be clear that I am referring to vertically integrated care, not horizontally integrated care. Integrated care refers to *a system that coordinates* all or much of the care a patient may need. Managed care is a *set of rules* about how care should be provided. Integrated systems often *use* managed care rules in delivering healthcare.

An example of an integrated *health plan* system would be one that contracts exclusively with one set of doctors and also exclusively with one set of hospitals, and those doctors and hospitals work closely together to make sure care for all their patients is coordinated. The system may, for example, set up automated connections for patients to get care at home following a hospitalization, and so on. An example of this type of integrated health plan is Kaiser Permanente, a large plan based in California with facilities in several states. Kaiser Permanente doctors, hospitals, and many other types of caregivers work in close cooperation with each other and use managed care rules in providing care to members. For example, a managed care rule used by the system might be that home care is provided following hospitalization only for specific types of surgeries or cases of a certain level of severity.

Other examples of integrated systems are when a medical group, separate from a health plan, works closely with a local hospital, also separate from a health plan, to set up coordinated systems of care for the group's patients. The doctors in this integrated arrangement may or may not use managed care rules, though it is rare these days to find systems that do not use managed care rules of some kind.

Three Signposts of Quality Integrated Care

The best integrated systems have the following traits in common.

1. Inclusivity: The Team Approach

Today's best integrated medical care systems provide and coordinate all outpatient and inpatient care as well as all support and ancillary services. These systems have teams that proactively set up services designed to anticipate your needs instead of just reacting to them when they occur. If your doctor participates in a good integrated system, he or she can connect you with many other professionals whose services might improve your health.

For example, your doctor would not only give you an authorization form for physical therapy, but would also connect you with a physical therapist. Your doctor would be part of an extensive closely connected team of providers, including physician specialists, health educators, case managers, and so forth—all of whom would work together to ensure that you get appropriate care. Such team arrangements work best when all parties work in one location and usually for one organization, as is the case for clinics. However, well-coordinated integrated systems could exist in non-clinic settings.

2. Top-Notch Care

The best integrated systems successfully implement the five elements of clinical quality. To recap, they are:

A. **Outcomes Measurement (See Chapter 9):** Top-quality integrated systems collect data on care *results*—how patients' health actually fared as a result of specific treatment. These results provide a basis for comparing care providers. They also enable the health plan to assess the effectiveness of both current treatments and improvement efforts.

B. Evidence-Based Treatment (See Chapter 10): When determining the best treatment for a patient, it is crucial that doctors use results of current and credible scientific studies rather than outdated medical school training, pharmaceutical promotional information, or chance discussions with colleagues. In the best systems, up-to-date treatment guidelines are readily available to providers. When new evidence comes to light, these systems implement the latest treatment recommendations quickly and systematically.

C. Avoidance of Medical Errors (See Chapter 11): Medical errors are prevalent nationwide. In the best systems, physicians and other caregivers acknowledge the importance of avoiding mistakes and strongly commit to reducing them. They do this by agreeing to practice rigorous honesty and by submitting to scrutiny their part in any error that occurs. Problems of poor coordination and miscommunication are reviewed constantly. Immediate action is taken to analyze and revamp systems and processes to avoid repeating errors.

D. Prevention (See Chapter 7): Focus on prevention of illness and the early treatment of disease is key. A good healthcare organization will not only give preventive tests and treatments but will also track what preventive care each patient still needs. It will also educate patients to become active in their own health promotion and to make healthful lifestyle changes. The best systems are proactive in encouraging members to get the preventive screening tests they need, instead of waiting for the member to make a checkup appointment. Doctors, receptionists, nurses, and other team members have systematic reminders that alert them each time they are involved with a patient in any way to arrange for the patient's specific prevention care.

E. Coordination of Care (See Chapter 12): The highest-quality healthcare organizations share and coordinate information among primary physicians, specialists, outpatient and inpatient care providers, and all ancillary services for each patient and for each episode of care or type of illness.

3. Quality Assurance Over Cost Saving

Excellent healthcare organizations do not emphasize revenue over quality of care. Some organizations develop innovative

> Today's best integrated medical care systems provide and coordinate all outpatient and inpatient care as well as all support and ancillary services.

ways to maximize the financial health of the organization while simultaneously providing high-quality care. Superior, forward-thinking healthcare systems all emphasize the following factors. Some of these add to the cost of care, at least short term, because they require additional investments into the system, but all improve the quality of care.

A. **Adherence to Performance Standards:** The highest-quality systems carefully scrutinize the competency, training, and conduct of physicians, nurses, and all other caregivers. Providers must meet high standards in all three of these areas to be accepted into the system. Caregivers with proven patterns of flagrant or repeated medical misconduct are excluded. Notably, good systems continue to review caregivers after their acceptance, and neither incompetence nor misconduct are tolerated among new or seasoned practitioners.

B. **Ongoing Commitment to Continuous Improvement:** High-achieving organizations commit on a system-wide basis to doing whatever it takes to provide *and continuously improve* quality of care. Management directives start at the top and reflect the intention to meet the highest quality standards. (Another way of saying this is that Quality is a key element in their business plan.)

   Committing to improving quality takes a great deal of courage and fortitude, because it means making changes in the way all participants do their day-to-day work. Change is never easy—for any of us.

C. **Investment in Data Collection and Communication Systems:** These organizations have also invested in data collection and communication systems. These systems are mostly, but not necessarily, large and comprehensive electronic programs. Of course, information technology plays a big part in these activities. Read more about healthcare's use of information technology in Chapter 16.

D. **Quality Improvement Through Innovation:** The best systems are developing new healthcare models that are more effective and/or more efficient. For example, some systems use group doctor visits, where sets of patients with a common illness can get the same treatment and disease management information. In addition to being more efficient than having each patient meet with the physician separately, patients benefit from hearing about the experiences of other patients who have the same health problems and who may have found good ways to cope.

Some systems implement effective new methods of electronic communication between doctors and their patients, such as having patients ask questions and get answers from their doctors on a secure Web page. Advanced systems are using home-based technology to communicate important information directly to doctors. A few systems use Internet-based platforms for patients to self-administer their risk-assessments, track personal medical information, and link to risk-management resources.

Excellent healthcare organizations do not emphasize revenue over quality of care.

Taking Integrated Care to Excellence

Coordination of care and quality assurance are not enough. Integrated organizations reach excellence only when they meet these further goals:

- Treat each patient as a full human being while systematizing care.

- Maintain a high level of service quality along with high clinical quality.

- Not get so bogged down in bureaucracy that the system becomes incapable of learning from its mistakes.

- Make it possible for physicians to maintain a high level of autonomy in their decision-making about treatments. Each of us is unique. Our medical problems don't always fit a standard pattern. Together with our doctors, we need to be able to customize our treatment plans.

Moving U.S. Medical Care Toward Integration

Steve Shortell, Dean of the School of Public Health, University of California at Berkeley, and his colleagues state in their most recent book,[2] "Implementing the promise of integrated healthcare will continue to be slow and uneven.....Almost everyone is playing around the edges...." Dr. Shortell predicts that the following five forces will push U.S. healthcare toward increased integration over the next 15 years:

1. An aging population. Many people over 65 have chronic illnesses. People with chronic diseases especially benefit from integrated systems of care. As the need to better manage chronic diseases in the most elderly part of the

population increases, healthcare will feel pressure to move more and more toward integration.

2. Technology. Accelerating developments in biomedical sciences, biotechnology, pharmaceuticals, and information technology will make it easier to improve healthcare using an integrated approach. Some of these new developments will make healthcare better by making it easier for patients to partner with physicians and other caregivers in managing their healthcare. Other developments will make it easier for health plans, medical groups, and individual physicians to give better care through improving the management of disease.

3. Empowered consumers. Aging baby boomers will likely demand a greater say in healthcare delivery. Consumers will increasingly seek out medical information online for choosing providers and for improving their care by partnering with their providers.

4. Payment innovations. Currently we do not pay physicians, hospitals, or other healthcare providers for providing well-integrated care, for good outcomes of care, or for improving health. We pay them for providing healthcare services, period. In fact, ironically, if the poor care you received causes you to need additional care, your providers get paid more than if you had received good care in the first place. If you develop an infection due to unclean conditions in a hospital, for example, the extra care you will need means the hospital will get paid for the extra services provided.

Current pay-for-performance movements in both the public (Medicare) and private sectors will create greater provider accountability. To be more accountable to payors, providers will need to develop more effective and efficient systems of care. This will lead to greater integration.

5. Ability to partner. The various parts of the healthcare industry are in many ways entrenched in their own worlds and find it challenging to partner with other parts of the industry. For example, doctors often are determined to remain independent of hospitals and health plans. Even though they are forced to interact with these other parts of the industry, doctors often do so as minimally as possible and with somewhat antagonistic attitudes. However, the four forces discussed briefly above will push all

parts of the industry toward better working partnerships so that together they can create better integrated care delivery systems. Those physicians, hospitals, health plans, and other parts of the industry best able to partner will most likely do best in the coming years.

16 Information: The Key to Effective Healthcare

The real voyage of discovery consists not of finding new lands but of seeing the territory with new eyes.

—Marcel Proust

In This Chapter...
- Many people have used the Internet as a source of information for health and medical information.
- More and more people will probably use the Internet as a source of information in the future.
- Email communication between doctors and patients will likely increase.
- Electronic communications have improved the administration of healthcare and will most likely continue to enhance administrative processes.
- Information technology has been slow to be adopted in the clinical aspects of healthcare.
- Technological processes envisioned for the future of medicine promise extraordinary improvements.

If you were asked what makes life different now from the way it was 50 years ago, or even 20 years ago, you might say that the biggest factor is the widespread and growing use of computers, or what is often called "Information Technology" (IT). IT includes using computers and the Internet to store, process, and distribute information and to assist in all kinds of mechanical and other activities. This phenomenon has an impact on almost every part of our lives and certainly on most industries in our economy. Though some people continue to argue the point, most agree that IT does improve our lives.

IT has already contributed greatly to healthcare. To give you a better understanding of how IT can improve things further, we will discuss four ways consumers interact with the healthcare industry.

Sources of Patient Information

The Internet

Harris Interactive recently conducted a large survey of consumer use of the Internet as a source of medical and health information.[1] The survey found that an estimated 109 million American adults, about 52% of the U.S. adult population, have looked for health information online. This represents about 80% of all American adults who have used the Internet for any reason. According to the Harris Interactive report, the percentage of American adults who have looked for health information online roughly doubled between 1998 and 2002, though the 2003 survey showed no significant change in the numbers over that year.

Another recent survey, conducted by the Pew Internet & American Life Project,[2] confirmed that 80% of adult American Internet users have looked for health or medical information online. The survey showed that people look for information to become informed, to prepare for appointments and surgery, to share information, and to look for and provide support.

Internet health information seekers also reported psychological and emotional benefits from this activity. They said they feel more in control and empowered by getting more information, often feel less alone by learning that many others share the same struggles, and feel less fear about their fates by gaining hope. The Pew survey showed that people who use the Internet to find health and medical information especially appreciate the anonymity they have in doing their search, the fact that they can access the Internet at any time of day or night, and the breadth of information they find. Eighty-two percent reported they were able to find what they were looking for "most of the time" or "always."

Three-fourths of these searchers reported that information gotten from the Internet improved the health information and services they received. They reported that some doctors were receptive to patient Internet research and some were not. Internet users also reported that they have difficulty finding the following types of information online and would like them to be more readily available or easier to find:

• Drug interactions

• Diagnostic tools or symptom finders

• Electronic medical records

- More information for caregivers
- More ways to connect with local resources
- Doctor-patient email
- More information on a doctor's background
- Better privacy protection
- Less spam, which can limit discussion on list-servs and bulletin boards
- Free access to medical journals containing important articles on diseases/conditions consumers are vitally interested in. Many full journal articles are available only to subscribers or to those able to pay a fee.

According to Kevin Fickenscher, MD, National Director and Partner for Clinical Transformation with Computer Sciences Corporation,[3] the medical data found on the Internet often provides only a basic understanding of the medical condition or treatment. In-depth information about symptoms, causes, and options for treatment and their pros and cons is rarely available.

if used wisely, the Internet may be the single best source of health and medical information for consumers.

There are four ways to use the Internet to find health information. I recommend the approach listed last below:

- Go directly to a known site. Many people know about sites such as WebMD, MSN Health, Yahoo!Health, and several other health information databases.

- Use search sites such as Google or Dogpile to find sites related to the search topic. For example, you might type "diabetes" as a topic at one of these search sites. The search would then bring up a long list of sites for you to choose from. Some sites will have trustworthy information and some will have inaccurate or biased information. Sorting through the list of sites is an inefficient way to find good medical information. According to a report by RAND Health prepared for the California Healthcare Foundation,[4] consumers using English search engines have only a one-in-five chance of finding what they need using this approach, and it takes a good deal of time. Using Spanish-language search engines gives even poorer results.

- Go to MEDLINE and search for published medical articles on your topic. The search function is easy at this site, and many of the articles found will contain very good information, especially those published in highly respected medical journals such as the *New England Journal of Medicine*. However, the articles are usually written for medical professionals and are often hard for the layperson to read and understand. In fact, even doctors not trained in the technicalities of high-level medical research sometimes misinterpret these research articles. You can easily print "abstracts" (brief summaries) of articles directly from the MEDLINE database when available (indicated by a special symbol beside the name of the article). When no abstract is available, you will most likely need to get a copy of the article from your public library, as many of these journals require a fee or a paid subscription to access the full article online.

> **Many problems of the U.S. healthcare system could be alleviated with better use of clinical informatics systems.**

• Use unbiased, prescreened, trustworthy sites such as those listed in Appendix A. I especially recommend MEDLINE-plus. You can use these sites to first get a high-level overview of your topic, then delve more deeply by going to other sites linked to or recommended by the main site.

In response to concern about the accuracy of medical information on the Internet, at least one trustworthy organization, URAC (which used to stand for Utilization Review Accreditation Commission but which is now just an acronym), recently began reviewing health information websites and accrediting those that pass scrutiny for accuracy. Also known as the American Accreditation Healthcare Commission, URAC is a non-profit organization that establishes standards for the healthcare industry. You can find URAC's list of approved websites at *www.urac.org*.

It is clear that there are pros and cons to accessing health and medical information on the Internet. Everything considered, however, and if used wisely, the Internet may be the single best source of health and medical information for consumers. Over time it may therefore be used more and more for this purpose. The benefits of the Internet make it far more useful for most people than relying on books and magazines for information.

Patient–Doctor Communication By Email

Traditionally, patients communicate with their doctors through face-to-face office visits or an occasional phone call. Often, doctors will not answer questions by phone, so patients are forced to make an office visit to get their medical questions answered.

Nowadays, some physicians are willing to converse with patients via email, especially with long-time patients whose health history and medical problems they know well. The benefit to the patient is time flexibility and the convenience of not having to go in for a visit. You can, for example, email your question at midnight when things are quiet for you and you have the chance to think through what you want to ask. Your doctor can respond when she or he has a free moment, and you can read the response in privacy whenever you choose. You also have a record of the response.

Recent surveys show that few doctors currently communicate with patients by email. Many say they prefer to speak to patients face-to-face, and others indicate that they might use email if they could be reimbursed for time spent at it. Few health plans currently reimburse doctors for email consultations, though some have recently started to do so.

Forty percent of consumers surveyed on this topic said they would be willing to pay for online doctor "visits." Potential problems with using the Internet for this purpose include privacy issues, but those who have tried this type of patient–doctor communication seem to have resolved these concerns.[5]

Long term, it seems likely that we will communicate with our doctors electronically more and more, and that we will all benefit from it. Later in this chapter you will find more ideas for using the Internet to interact with your doctor.

Information Technology in Administration

Almost all health plans and insurance companies have been working to make their administrative processes more efficient by implementing new computerized systems. Most of these improvements benefit consumers, either directly or indirectly. Faster verification of patient eligibility, reduced cycle times for claims payments, and faster referral and service preauthorization are some of the improvements that have been achieved.

Numerous health plans now have websites where members can check the status of their claims payments. Administrative process improvements also reduce the total costs of healthcare. Since both providers and consumers are unhappy about the current level of administrative hassles they endure, we can hope that many more improvements are in the works.

Clinical Informatics Systems for Improved Care

Compared to other U.S. industries, healthcare has been slow to implement information technology. Although the insurance companies and doctors' offices have used IT systems for billing and administrative functions for some time now, IT

Clinical informatics systems can create reminders for physicians, such as reminders to prescribe appropriate preventive care or reminders of care guidelines for specific diagnoses based on the latest scientific evidence.

systems for helping doctors practice medicine (called clinical informatics systems) are new.

Many problems of the U.S. healthcare system could be alleviated with better use of clinical informatics systems. Examples include poorly coordinated care, doctors forgetting to prescribe preventive care, doctors unable to keep up with the latest scientific research, medical errors, and so on.

Some doctors in larger medical groups have already implemented clinical informatics systems or are in the process of doing so. However, these systems are expensive, and doctors have little incentive to incur the costs they require. In other words, doctors do not get paid more, do not get more patients, nor do they benefit financially in any other way for improving how they practice medicine.

This is one instance where we as consumers can take action to significantly improve the quality of medical care in the U.S. Doctors who use good patient data information tracking systems generally provide higher-quality care than those who do not.[6] It just makes sense that using electronic systems is the best and most efficient way to track data. This should steer you toward those physicians who use clinical informatics systems. If enough of us leave our non-technologically-savvy physicians and start choosing those who use the best technology to improve our care, then those physicians resisting this change will be forced to rethink their position.

It is unfortunate that the latest technologies require a costly investment from physicians. However, just about every other industry has had to face the same challenge to stay competitive. The Institute of Medicine has proposed that the federal government provide financial aid to physicians to improve their clinical IT capabilities. This proposal is based on the now firmly established link between the use of these systems and an improvement in quality of care.[7]

How do the new clinical informatics systems help doctors do their work? Here's a good example. Some systems create an electronic medical record for each patient, eliminating the traditional use of paper records. Tracking each patient's medical information electronically means, among other things, that multiple members of your healthcare team can access the record at any time. It eliminates the problem of your information being unavailable to one member of the team because your chart is sitting on another team member's desk.

If the system is designed well, it also means that your doctor can easily find important information in your records that may be difficult to find in a paper chart, especially if you have a large chart due to many medical problems. For example, lab test results are often easier to find and track in an electronic record than in a paper chart.

Here's another example of how doctors can use this powerful technology to improve the care they provide. Clinical informatics systems can create reminders for physicians, such as reminders to prescribe appropriate preventive care or reminders of care guidelines for specific diagnoses based on the latest scientific evidence. For example, there are many components to giving the best care to diabetics. Doctors treating diabetic patients need a systematic way to collect and track multiple types of information about each patient. They also need a system that reminds them to do all the things each diabetic patient needs done. A clinical informatics system can provide this kind of help.

Information Technology: Present & Future

Healthcare IT experts have thought a great deal about how to improve healthcare using the best technology available. What they envision is a utopia that would be astounding. Kevin Fickenscher, MD, of Computer Sciences Corp. (mentioned earlier), is one of these visionaries. Information in this section comes from his work.

To give you a mental picture of what Dr. Fickenscher envisions, here are two tales. The first takes place in the year 2000; the second in 2010.

Tale No. 1: The Saga of Mr. Smykowski, circa 2000
This tale shows how things happen today.

• Two weeks ago, Mr. Smykowski visited his doctor, Dr. Monto, for a regular checkup. Dr. Monto's office staff checked Mr. Smykowski's blood pressure, and the results showed his blood pressure was high. Dr. Monto suspected that Mr. Smykowski's cholesterol and blood glucose levels might also be high, based on Mr. Smykowski's family history, and so Dr. Monto ordered lab tests to confirm. Because Mr. Smykowski gets little to no exercise, is overweight, and has smoked a pack-and-a-half of cigarettes each day for the past 23 years, Dr. Monto told Mr. Smykowski that he is a prime candidate for heart disease. However, Mr. Smykowski's routine EKG test, performed that day in the doctor's office, was normal, giving no indication of any problems. The next day, Mr. Smykowski went to the lab for the tests Dr. Monto had ordered.

The chart below reflects Mr. Smykowski's initial interaction with the healthcare system. As the stars in the chart show, he connected with two parts of the system: his physician and the lab.

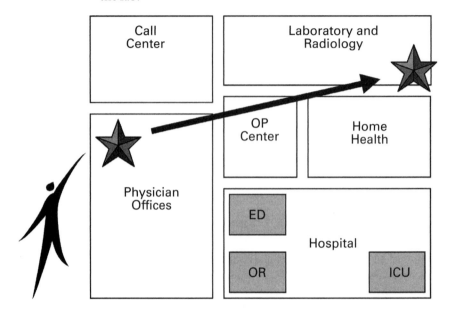

- On a Sunday afternoon at about 2:00 p.m., just after eating a big meal at his mother's house, Mr. Smykowski begins to have what feels like severe digestive distress. After taking some antacid and suffering mightily for awhile, he calls his health plan's call center to ask what he should do. The call center nurse tells him if it does not get better soon he should go to the nearest emergency room.

- Six hours later Mr. Smykowski still feels a great deal of discomfort and goes to the emergency room, telling the ER doctor he "must have eaten something bad."

The chart on the following page shows Mr. Smykowski's continuing interaction with the healthcare system. As the stars in the chart now show, he has connected with four parts of the system: his physician, the lab, his health plan's call center, and the hospital emergency room.

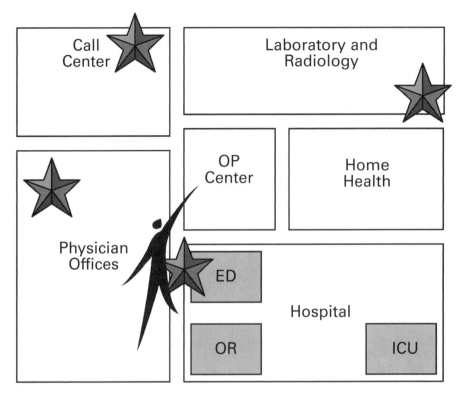

- The attending ER doctor determines that Mr. Smykowski is showing signs of having a heart attack, so he contacts Dr. Monto. The ER physician also calls a cardiologist in for a consultation.

- The ER doctor also arranges for Mr. Smykowski to immediately have an emergency angiogram. In preparation for the angiogram, the ER doctor orders the same lab work that had been done on Mr. Smykowski on an ambulatory basis. The angiogram reveals a major blockage in one of Mr. Smykowski's coronary arteries.

- Mr. Smykowski is immediately sent to the operating room for triple bypass surgery and then to the intensive care unit for recovery.

- Dr. Monto then finally gets the results of the lab tests done two weeks ago, which reveal high cholesterol and glucose levels.

- When Dr. Monto meets with Mr. Smykowski shortly after Mr. Smykowski's release from the hospital, the hospital record has not yet been transcribed and is not available. Dr.

Monto is not able to review the recommendations of the cardiologist called in for consultation or the cardiologist's follow-up lab orders. Dr. Monto prescribes smoking cessation classes, a weight loss program, an exercise program, and a cardiac support group program.

The chart below again shows Mr. Smykowski's continuing interaction with the healthcare system. As the stars in the chart now show, he has connected with six parts of the system: his physician, the lab, his health plan's call center, the emergency room, the operating room, and the intensive care unit.

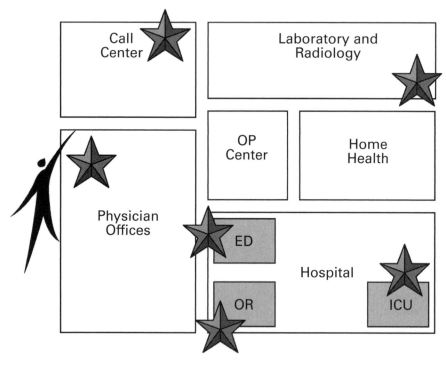

Let's assess services provided for Mr. Smykowski:
No or little physician office information is available outside of the 8-5 time period.

Call centers do not have access to provider-focused information.

Test results and other reporting are frequently delayed.

Cost of care is increased because of repeat testing and procedures.

Delays occur in the delivery of care because of a lack of information.

The patient is forced to provide the same information repeatedly at each point of care.

Tale No. 2: The Saga of Mr. S (Mr. Smykowski's Younger Brother), circa 2010

This tale shows how things might happen in the future. The doctor's office is electronically connected to all critical parts of the system. The doctor's office is connected to the hospital on a real-time basis 24/7. Lab and x-ray results are dynamically available. (That is, as soon as a test is completed, the test results are available to everyone in all other parts of the system.) Internal systems within the confines of the hospital are totally integrated. For example, the lab connects to the operating room scheduling, which connects to the intensive care unit management.

- Mr. S begins to have what feels like severe digestive distress.

- Mr. S logs onto AOL for advice on digestion problems but is not satisfied.

- Mr. S logs onto Dr. Monto's Web page and answers a series of questions about his health, which automatically updates his office medical record. Based on his responses to the questions and a review of the medical record, the software automatically allows Mr. S to schedule an appointment.

- Mr. S's demographic information and other personal data that his physician might want to know, including how much exercise he is currently getting and how many cigarettes he smokes daily currently and historically, is kept in a secure spot on the Internet. Mr. S has made this information accessible to his doctor. Mr. S checks to make sure his demographic and other information is up-to-date to save his doctor time in making a diagnosis.

- Mr. S sees his doctor in the office visit that was scheduled via the Internet. The office staff checks Mr. S's blood pressure. The results are high. The doctor suspects Mr. S's cholesterol and blood glucose levels might also be high given his family history. Mr. S's brother was seen on an emergency basis about 10 years ago with similar findings. Dr. Monto writes orders for lab tests to confirm. Because Mr. S gets little to no exercise, is overweight, and has been smoking for many years, Dr. Monto tells him he is a prime candidate for heart disease. However, Mr. S's routine EKG test, performed that day in the doctor's office, is normal, giving no indication of any current problem. Mr. S is reassured. The next day, Mr. S goes to the lab for the tests his doctor has ordered.

• Two weeks later, Mr. S again feels severe digestive distress. His older brother insists that he call his health plan's call center immediately to ask what he should do. Because Mr. S has given prior permission, all of his records are immediately available to the call center nurse, who tells him to go to the emergency room immediately.

The chart below shows Mr. S's initial interaction with the healthcare system. The solid and dotted lines show real-time dynamic availability of all data to all three parts of the system he has touched so far.

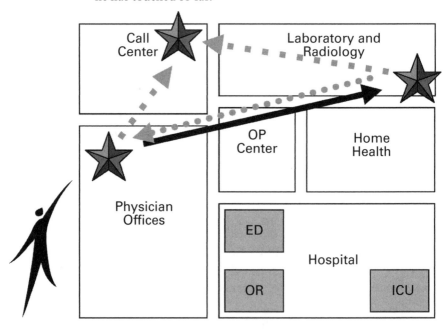

• Upon entering the ER, the following things automatically happen:

• Mr. S's doctor, Dr. Monto, is electronically paged.

• All information from prior visits, including lab test results, is immediately available to all caregivers in all parts of the system.

• The cardiologist preferred by Dr. Monto is contacted for a consultation.

• An angiogram, ordered immediately, reveals blockage of

a major artery. Lab tests do not need to be repeated to prepare for the angiogram because the results of the tests done two weeks previously were available in the patient's electronic medical record.

- Mr. S is immediately sent to the operating room for a combined triple laser procedure and genetic manipulation (for preventive purposes).

- An embedded chip is implanted (with Mr. S's permission) to monitor the hemodynamic status of his coronary arteries.

- The data on Mr. S's condition is submitted to a special "intelligent" data repository for meta-analysis of his situation and recommended course.

- Post-recovery plans include:

- Smoking cessation classes initiated with Web support

- Weight loss program

- Exercise program

- Cardiac support program with Web support services

- Continuous feedback and monitoring of participation in all initiatives

- Daily feedback from the internal chip monitors Mr. S's heart health status

- Mr. S has a follow-up appointment with Dr. Monto.

- The hospital record is available, including data from all tests, recommendations from the cardiologist, and orders for follow-up lab tests.

- Exercise and smoking cessation compliance data is available.

- Websites used by Mr. S are part of the care audit, including questions from Mr. S's wife.

The chart below shows Mr. S's continuing interaction with the healthcare system. The lines show a dynamic sharing of data among all parts of the system.

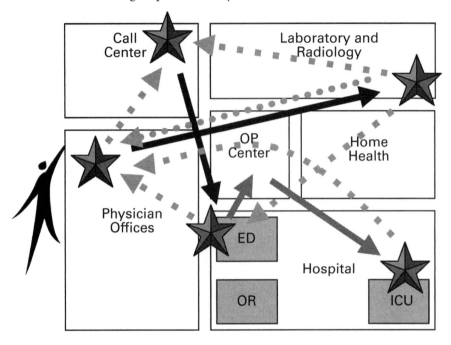

Let's assess services provided for Mr. S:

Physician office information is available 24/7 from any computer with a browser.

Call centers have full access to provider-focused information—intelligent software assists nurses in making recommendations for care.

Test results and other reporting are integrated into the data sharing systems as soon as the results are available.

Cost of care is reduced because repeat testing and procedures are eliminated.

Delivery of appropriate care is accelerated because of the availability of pertinent information.

The patient provides personal demographic data only once.

The Best-Case Scenario

For total information integration, all players in the system must be linked. The diagram below illustrates this concept. The scenario about Mr. S shows how the patient, the physician, the health plan's call center, and several units of the hospital could be linked electronically to share data in a beneficial way. Ideally, all other parts of healthcare would be linked with these parts also.

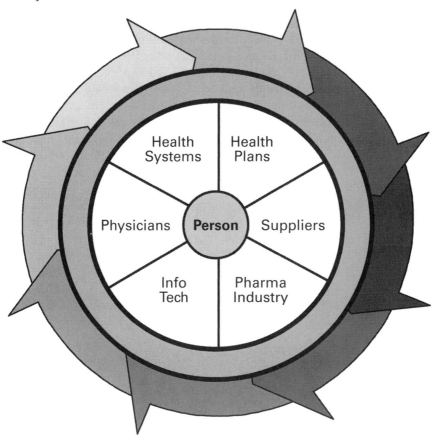

As the diagram indicates, the person receiving care must be at the center of this sharing of data. Privacy concerns would be built into this utopian arrangement. The patient would need to give permission to share his or her personal data with each link in the system, and all links would provide secure protection to prevent leakage of the data to anyone not authorized by the patient to have it.

Additional links to other parts of healthcare, such as to the health plan's administration system, would maximize the plan's ability to provide additional, personalized, useful services to the patient, such as information about smoking cessation class dates, times, and locations nearest to the patient's home. Links to the pharmaceutical industry could provide personalized messages to the patient and doctor with a link to websites where the patient could read about all prescribed medications. And so on.

How Close to Best-Case Are We?

The improvements in the quality of care envisioned in the tale of Mr. S are significant. According to a recent survey, most American consumers would like to see even more spent on healthcare as the economy grows.[8] Given this desire and the willingness to pay, and provided the economy does grow, we will most likely soon see some of these envisioned advances.

One recent development gives even more hope. In November 2003, the Institute of Medicine (IOM) issued a report calling for all hospitals and physicians to implement electronic patient record-keeping systems. The systems described by IOM can guide treatment decisions and catch mistakes, thus giving clear quality-of-care advantages. According to the report, eventually doctors and hospitals will need to have electronic patient record systems that meet government standards in order to be reimbursed through Medicare and other government programs. When this reimbursement requirement is established, the systems will essentially become a mandatory cost of doing business.[9]

PART V
WHICH TYPE OF PLAN TO CHOOSE?

U.S. consumers face a bewildering array of health plans to choose from. Part V discusses the major types of plans, pointing out the pros and cons and essential differences or similarities among them.

My goal here is to impart more in-depth information than consumers normally receive about the various health plan types. You will learn why the cost and quality may differ, sometimes greatly, among plan types. Partly because this topic is complex, there is little information about it available to the public.

This knowledge can help you choose the health plan that will be best for you. It can also help you understand and handle any problems you may have as a patient and/or claims-payer in a particular type of plan.

Whatever choices you make, you won't regret the time and energy you spend studying your options. A knowledgeable consumer is a wise consumer, and in the case of healthcare, a wise consumer is bound to be a healthier one too.

17 Indemnity Plans

Money is the last enemy that shall never be subdued. While there is flesh there is money—or the want of money, but money is always on the brain so long as there is a brain in reasonable order.
—Samuel Butler

In This Chapter...
A description of several aspects of indemnity plans and a chart that summarizes them.

Background

Let's start with indemnity plans, since they were the first and most straightforward of the health insurance plans widely available. Indemnity plans were created after World War II, during a period in which the U.S. government was imposing a national salary freeze. Companies found that adding healthcare benefits was a way to give their employees something extra without violating the wage freeze.

In an indemnity plan, the insurance company charges a premium, usually on a monthly basis, and reimburses patients for covered services after the patient has paid the provider and submitted a claim. (Sometimes the provider is willing to bill the insurance company and be paid directly for the amount covered, charging the patient only for the non-covered portion of the bill.) Reimbursement is based on a fee-for-service arrangement. In other words, when a doctor provides a service—an office visit, for example—he or she charges the patient a specified amount of money (a fee) in exchange for that service.

A big drawback to many indemnity plans is that they often do not cover preventive care. The reason is that these plans were designed primarily to protect against the high financial costs of catastrophic health events. They were not designed to assist people with day-to-day healthcare costs.

How Patients Get Care

Using an indemnity plan is pretty straightforward. Customers can go to any physician or hospital they choose, without any restrictions. No referral is required to see a specialist. The insurance company has no say over what the doctor can or cannot do in treating the patient. As long as the type of service provided is covered under the policy, the customer (or the provider) is reimbursed for the covered portion of the fee with no questions asked. However, in indemnity plans that include a Utilization Review component, nonemergency hospitalization and certain outpatient procedures require the health plan's prior approval in order to be covered by the policy.

A big drawback to many indemnity plans is that they often do not cover preventive care.

How Providers Are Paid

As we have discussed, providers (doctors, hospitals, and all other caregivers) are paid a fee for each service they provide (called "fee-for-service").

Financial Forces Impacting Your Care

Financial motivations drive the care given by many providers. The goal is to give as much care as possible and charge as much as the market will bear per service so as to increase provider income. Providers tend to feel that since the insurance company (or the government in the case of Medicare) is paying the bill, they may as well get as much as possible. This can lead to patients being given some treatments they may not need, or at least that are questionably necessary. Another inclination related to fee-for-service is for providers to cater to and focus on illness care rather than on care that will keep patients well. Preventive care provides minimal reimbursement to the doctor. Sick patients bring in more money to the physician than well patients do, especially when income per minute of work is considered.

The desire to help every patient gives good doctors an incentive to get you the care you need, either preventive or illness care. However, human nature being what it is, the financial motivations are bound to have an impact on many, if not on most, physicians.

Quality

Quality varies—a lot. The insurance company has absolutely no control over the quality of care provided in an indemnity plan.

Costs

As stated above, under the fee-for-service payment method the financial incentive for doctors and hospitals is to provide as many services as possible and charge as much as possible in order to maximize their income. As a result of this payment arrangement, the costs of indemnity coverage are the highest of all plan types. This is true even in those indemnity plans with a Utilization Review component, which controls costs to some degree.

Financial motivations drive the care given by many providers.

Pros

Patients have a great deal of freedom in choosing doctors and hospitals. Other than the requirement to obtain preauthorization for specified types of high-cost care where there is a Utilization Review component, patients are not saddled with a lot of rules and regulations for getting care.

Cons

Understanding what a policy covers can be daunting. Submission and processing of claim forms are tedious and often confusing, and can involve a great deal of time to keep things sorted out with the insurance company. Preventive care is not covered in many indemnity plans. There is absolutely no control over quality except where the Utilization Review component determines whether a requested procedure is appropriate and necessary.

Indemnity Plan—Summary

Overall Value

• Not a good value.

• Provides the ultimate level of choice since you can use any provider, but the lack of cost controls make indemnity coverage extremely expensive.

• The consumer must assume total responsibility for finding high-quality care because indemnity plans do not participate in quality comparison surveys.

Clinical Quality

(–) No guarantee of quality. Choose MD, medical group, and hospital carefully—based on quality reviews and surveys when available.

Ease of Getting Care

(+) Since you can use any MD and any hospital, you do not have the hassle of figuring out which MDs are on the health plan's "list."

(–) Frustrating amounts of paperwork are often required for claims-filing.

Costs

(–) Fee-for-service can provide an incentive for MDs to prescribe more care than is necessary.

(–) Most expensive of all plan types.

(–) Preventive care must often be paid for entirely by the patient, in addition to the high costs of the coverage.

18 HMOs

Error of opinion may be tolerated where reason is left free to combat it. —Thomas Jefferson

In This Chapter...
A description of several aspects of Health Maintenance Organization (HMO) plans and a chart that summarizes them.

Background

The Health Maintenance Organization or HMO was initially called a "prepaid group practice plan." These plans were created as early as the 1800s in a variety of small communities across the U.S., mostly to serve populations of workers who might otherwise not be able to afford medical care (i.e., iron miners in Minnesota, pineapple plantation workers in Hawaii, lumberjacks in Oregon and Washington, Henry Kaiser's water project, and shipyard workers in California and Oregon).

The distinguishing feature of these plans was that all care was provided in exchange for prepaid monthly membership "dues." These prepayments set a firm budget within which the plan doctors had to do all of their work—quite different from the prevailing standard of "fee-for-service" medicine where physicians could charge for every service they provided.[1]

As discussed in Chapter 17, fee-for-service payment mechanisms to doctors (in indemnity plans and other types of plans we will discuss) create an incentive for doctors to provide as many services as possible, whether they are needed or not. Fee-for-service creates a focus on disease rather than a focus on health, since unhealthy patients need more care (and thus provide more income to the physician) than healthy ones do. Preventive care is relatively inexpensive to provide and does not get the physician reimbursed at very high levels under fee-for-service.

In contrast, the major financial incentive created in HMOs was to keep members as healthy as possible (thus the name "health maintenance") in order to avoid having to provide care for preventable medical problems—thereby saving overall costs. The second most important incentive in HMOs was to provide services as efficiently as possible, since all care had to be provided within the preset budget. This, too, was quite a contrast to fee-for-service.

By 1970, there were 33 HMOs in the U.S. with a total of 3 million members. During the 1980s the federal government promoted and supported the development of additional plans. The idea was to combat the rising costs of indemnity insurance. The government recognized that the dramatically increasing costs of indemnity health plans were a direct result of the skyrocketing fees charged by providers being reimbursed by fee-for-service arrangements.

Under HMOs, enrollees generally are able to get better coverage for less money than under the indemnity plans. As the costs of indemnity coverage continued to escalate, consumers were encouraged to enroll in HMOs. By 1996, there were almost 600 HMOs with a total of 60 million members. This was nearly 20 times as many HMOs as in 1970, with a 2,000% increase in membership! Membership in HMOs increased throughout the 1990s, but began to decline after the late 1990s due to member frustration at difficulty getting care in HMOs.

How Patients Get Care

Each HMO has a specific set of contracted doctors, hospitals, and other care providers. Members must use these providers in order for the plan to cover their care. Some HMO plans have exclusive contractual arrangements with a single physician group. Doctors in this group do not treat anyone except members of that HMO and, conversely, members are required to see only that group's doctors. Other HMOs have doctors on their list who take patients from more than one HMO. Many HMOs require each member to choose a family doctor (referred to as the member's Primary-Care Physician or PCP). In these plans, the PCP manages all of the member's care. Keep reading for more explanation of the different types of HMOs.

Group-Model HMOs

Under the *group-model HMO*, the physician group is a legally separate organization that contracts only with one health plan, which is the "insurance" part of the HMO. One example of this arrangement is the Permanente Medical Groups, which contract exclusively with Kaiser Foundation Health Plans to provide care to Kaiser's 9 million members in 16 states.

Staff-Model HMOs

Under the *staff-model HMO*, the doctors are salaried employees of the health plan. They are not employees of the medical group, as in group-model plans. Doctors in a staff-model HMO do not have their own legally separate organization. This difference between group- and staff-model HMOs is one that even knowledgeable insiders get confused about. The differences may seem subtle but are significant to the participating doctors.

Group- and staff-model HMOs sometimes own and operate their own hospitals, though some contract with independent hospitals in addition to or instead of having their own.

Network-Model HMOs

Another type of HMO is the *network-model HMO*—where independent physicians, physician groups, and hospitals contract with a health plan to treat the consumers enrolled in that plan. The independent physicians, physician groups, and hospitals often contract with more than one health plan. For example, ABC Medical Group may have HMO contracts with Aetna, Health Net, and Blue Cross, and the doctors in that medical group may treat HMO members from each of these insurance carriers—in addition to PPO and indemnity plan members.

Looking at the health plan side of the equation, each of the health plans usually has contracts with multiple medical groups and hospitals. Each health plan's network may overlap the other health plans' networks to some degree, but usually not entirely. For example, Aetna, Health Net, and Blue Cross may have Hospitals W and X on their lists, with Hospital Y being on Aetna's and Blue Cross's lists but not on the Health Net list, and Hospital Z being on Aetna's list but not on any others. This pattern applies to medical groups as well as hospitals.

When a physician group or a set of physicians affiliate with a single health plan, as in group- and staff-model plans, cooperation and collaboration between the physicians and the health plan is much easier than when each physician must work with multiple health plans. However, the network-model plan usually offers consumers a broader choice of doctors and hospitals. This ability to offer greater choice of providers is the reason there are far more network-model HMOs than group- or staff-model plans. As we've discussed in previous chapters, consum-

> Under HMOs, enrollees generally are able to get better coverage for less money than under the indemnity plans.

Health Plan Hassles

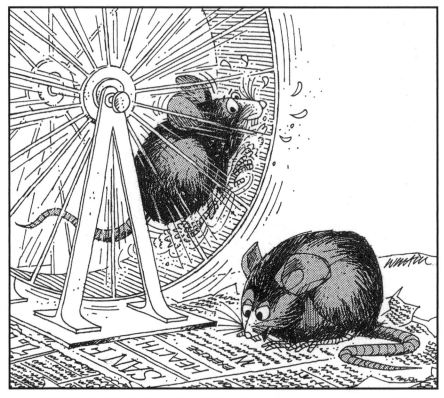

"IT SAYS HERE YOU HAVE TO RUN BACKWARDS THEN FORWARDS THREE TIMES TO GET TO SEE A SPECIALIST."

ers tend to prefer plans with more choice. (Remember, however, that greater choice of provider does not guarantee higher quality. Higher quality can be had under restricted choice situations, as long as the restricted choices are good ones.)

How Providers Are Paid

HMO doctors are often paid on a per-head basis, meaning the doctor is paid a set amount of money each month for each member assigned to him or her, regardless of how many or what types of services are needed. (For those of you who like to know such things, this is called "capitation.") Sometimes it is the primary-care physician (PCP) who receives this per-patient money from the health plan each month. Then, in turn, the PCP pays specialists to whom he or she refers patients. More often, this set amount of money per member per month is paid to the PCP's medical group, which then pays each participating doctor, including primary-care and specialist physicians, according to the amount of time and care they have put in for all the medical group's patients.

Under this basis for compensation, the medical group gets paid even for members who never use services. However, the medical group must cover costs of providing care to all assigned members, even the sickest ones who require more than average care. Thus the financial risk for the doctors is "spread" across many patients. If payments are not adequate to cover all of the services needed by a set of patients (perhaps because many are more ill than average), doctors can lose money.

However, if this monthly payment amount is set at the right level, this payment method encourages doctors to provide all appropriate preventive screening and exactly the right amount of necessary care for each patient. Giving more than necessary care would bust the budget. Providing less than necessary care is avoided because it will ultimately lead to providing more care as the patient gets sicker after the illness is not arrested in its early stages.

Many doctors claim they are not being paid enough under their HMO contracts. As a result, many have either refused to contract with HMOs at all or are dropping their HMO affiliations. Interestingly, this appears to be much less of a problem in group- and staff-model HMOs. There are far more instances of doctors dropping out of network-model HMOs in which solo physicians and/or physician groups tend to contract with multiple health plans. Physicians seem to be happier in group- and staff-model HMOs at least partly because they have more and better resources to support them—even though they are receiving roughly the same take-home pay as network-model HMO doctors—and because they don't have to deal with the multiple sets of rules of multiple health plans, and they don't have to run a business. They just get to take care of patients.

Because of this per-member, per-month type of payment arrangement, most network-model HMOs must require each member to choose a primary-care physician. The member must use only one PCP during a specified month. If the patient wishes to switch PCPs, this must be done at the beginning of a month and is effective for the entire month. Otherwise the health plan would not know to which medical group to pay the monthly capitation payment. As another result of this capitation payment arrangement, the specialist used by a network-model HMO member must belong to the same medical group as the PCP. Otherwise the specialist cannot be paid because his or her payment is tied to the monthly payment made to the PCP.

> Many HMOs now allow direct access to some or all specialists without getting a referral from your PCP.

Financial Forces Impacting Your Care

To summarize, the financial incentives for the healthcare provider paid on a per-head basis are:

- Keep patients as healthy as possible to avoid having to treat preventable illness. This means giving patients appropriate preventive care and counseling for a healthful lifestyle. Please note it does not mean giving preventive care that has not been proven effective nor giving checkups more often than have shown to be necessary.

- Provide care as efficiently as possible. This means that office visits are as short as possible, appointments may be difficult to get for non-urgent care, unneeded care will not be authorized, and questionably needed care may be denied. Controversies arise fairly often, both between the doctor and the health plan and between patients and their doctors, about what is and what is not necessary care. These discussions are appropriate as long as patient, physician, and health plan are acting as responsible partners and as long as all sides are armed with accurate facts. Sometimes it is not easy to figure out exactly what care is or is not necessary. Open discussions between knowledgeable doctors helps in finding the best answers, though many doctors seem uncomfortable with this process.

Another result of practicing medicine as efficiently as possible is that your PCP, usually a family doctor, may insist on providing treatment that you might have gone to a specialist to receive. This is often a less costly way to give you the care you need. This practice has potential pros and cons for a patient. It is good for the patient when the PCP's treatment is as effective as the treatment you would have received from the specialist. It is not a good thing when the care you receive from the PCP is less effective than the care the specialist would have provided. Unfortunately, most patients don't know the types of care their primary doctor gives that are just as good as a specialist would give. This is one instance where arming yourself with information on best practices, by looking up the science-based guidelines for the treatment of your illness, can really help you. The information you gather can serve as the basis for a discussion with your doctor.

Ease of Getting Care

Research shows that many HMO members have the following types of problems,[2] which usually have more to do with the process of getting care than with the quality of care received.

- Difficulty getting referrals to see specialists and authorizations to receive certain treatments.

- Frustration when their prescription drug coverage is changed.

- Confusion about emergency coverage.

- Poor understanding of how to resolve problems.

Other research, done at the University of California, Berkeley,[3] found differences in the experiences of members of network-model HMOs versus those in one very large group-model HMO. The major difference between the two was the degree to which services were integrated. The group-model HMO owns its infrastructure, including its hospitals and medical offices. All care for enrolled members is provided and coordinated within that infrastructure. Also, group-model doctors work only with that one health plan. Members of this group-model HMO tended to have fewer complaints than members of the network-model plans, even fewer than survey participants who were members of PPOs.

A recent survey done by Consumers Union and reported in *Consumer Reports* indicates that people enrolled in HMOs versus those enrolled in PPOs have similar levels of satisfaction, except those with back pain and arthritis, who prefer PPOs. Billing and customer service satisfaction was higher in

HMOs. Most importantly, those enrolled in the highest-rated HMOs were significantly more satisfied than those enrolled in the lowest-rated HMOs.[4]

The Gatekeeper Function

Some HMOs designate the PCP as the "gatekeeper" for all care given to members assigned to that PCP. This means that your PCP must authorize and make arrangements for all care you receive. If you need to see a specialist, you must get a referral from your PCP. And remember, unless an exception is made under unusual circumstances, the specialist must be a part of your PCP's medical group. If you need any tests, procedures, or surgery, all must be approved and arranged by your PCP. This gatekeeper arrangement is designed to serve as follows:

- **As a budget-control mechanism.** Since the doctor or his/her medical group is receiving only so much money for your care every month, someone must manage that money to make sure it will cover your care needs and leave the right amount for the doctor's income.

- **As a quality-control mechanism.** By limiting the source of member care, it is possible for health plans to measure the quality of care members receive. The PCP's medical group has all records of your care, so someone can check those records to verify the quality of care given to you. By measuring and comparing the level of quality you receive, the HMO can hold your PCP accountable for quality. In contrast, if you have totally free choice of physicians, there is no contract through which physicians can be held accountable for quality. When consumers have the freedom to use any doctor at any time, multiple PCPs and specialists from multiple medical groups may be used. This makes linking health results to care provided by a specific doctor or medical group nearly impossible.

Many HMOs now allow direct access to some or all specialists without getting a referral from your PCP. However, the specialist you see must still usually be part of the same medical group as your PCP in order for your care to be covered by the plan.

Costs

Total costs of care in HMOs tend to be less than costs for other types of plans. Total costs tend to be slightly higher in network-model HMO plans than in group- and staff-model plans. The efficiency of the highly integrated group- and staff-model plans provide the cost savings.

> By finding and using a highly rated HMO plan, you can get the best value available in U.S. healthcare.

Quality

Public consensus is that HMOs are bad news. The good news—mostly not understood by the public—is that quality of care in HMOs is easier to measure than in other types of plans. Therefore it is easier to control and improve. As previously discussed, this is because care can be more easily tracked. Patients' records are all in one place, and quality measurements can be built into contracts with participating doctors. When quality is measured, improvements can be insisted upon and measured. When quality is not measured, everyone is operating in the dark, including the doctors.

Choosing Physicians

Another aspect of HMO quality that consumers need to know about is how HMOs choose their participating physicians and hospitals. HMO strategies and processes for this vary greatly. Some HMOs simply accommodate the public's preference for having many choices of providers. These HMOs invite all local providers to be on their list, without quality discrimination, as long as the providers accept the HMO's fees. The HMOs that provide the highest quality of care, however, have very high standards for the physicians and hospitals they accept. This may mean that their list is short but excellent. On the other hand, a short list may instead mean that few local providers care to be part of that HMO because of the HMO's reputation for poor quality. It is important for you to find out how an HMO chooses its providers. If available, find quality surveys showing results for the medical groups on the HMO's list.

Pros

By finding and using a highly rated HMO plan, you can get the best value available in U.S. healthcare. With highly integrated HMO systems, you also get the convenience of having all services in more-or-less one geographic location. You often get added resources such as nurse-advice lines that are highly coordinated with all other services and low-cost, easily accessible health education classes on a wide variety of topics.

Another advantage of choosing a highly rated HMO is that the plan's financial incentives and systems are designed to keep you healthy and detect/treat illness early. These goals align with your need to stay as healthy as possible.

Cons

The financial incentives of capitation payment systems create a strong push to stay within a tightly set budget. This can make providers inclined to skimp on care. This inclination becomes especially strong when physicians are pushed to be highly productive, thus keeping appointments as short as possible. It is up to every patient to make sure he or she is getting all needed care, including getting all questions answered.

In some HMO plans, members experience frustrations when trying to get care. Rules for seeing specialists, for example, can be cumbersome. This is truer in network-model plans than in group- and staff-model plans.

You must use the plan's doctors and hospitals. This can be good or bad, depending on the level of quality provided by these doctors and hospitals.

If changing to an HMO means you must change doctors, this can be a hassle until you find and become established in your relationship with the new doctor.

HMO—Summary

Overall Value

• HMO plans that rate highly in legitimate quality surveys and have good prices compared to other choices are excellent values.

• Look for plans that rate highly in the surveys in both clinical quality and patient satisfaction.

Clinical Quality

(+) In many HMOs, data is collected to measure certain aspects of quality. If an HMO participates in a quality survey, its quality of care can be compared to that of other HMOs.

(+) HMO MDs and hospitals can be held accountable for measuring and improving quality.

(−) Some HMOs emphasize cost-control over quality.

(−) There is no guarantee of quality. Choose your health plan, MD, and hospital carefully.

Ease of Getting Care

(+) In staff/group HMOs, getting care is often very convenient. Because the plan directly provides all care, it often places its pharmacies, labs, and other services in the same location as its doctors' offices.

(−) In network-model HMOs, you must visit multiple locations to get all of your services.

(−) Some HMOs still require that you be referred by your PCP to any specialist you need to see. In essentially all cases, the specialist you see must be in the PCP's medical group. The referral process can be cumbersome. Check consumer satisfaction ratings of any plan you are considering joining.

(+) No claim forms need to be submitted except for out-of-plan emergency care.

Costs

(+) When the amount of coverage and total out-of-pocket costs are considered, HMOs are generally the least-expensive types of health plans.

19 PPOs

When a fellow says it ain't the money but the principle of the thing, it's the money. —Kin Hubbard

In This Chapter...
A description of many aspects of PPO plans and a chart that summarizes them.

Background

The Preferred Provider Organization ("PPO") came into being during the 1980s—about the same time as the number of HMOs drastically increased. PPOs were created as a compromise between the fee-for-service system, in which there was essentially no management of care by the insurance company, and HMOs, in which care was heavily managed. PPOs were created to be a "managed care lite" approach to healthcare.

As HMOs have gained a growing reputation for making it difficult to obtain needed care, PPOs have become more popular because they put fewer restrictions on how you receive care and which providers you can use. While HMOs will not pay for any care received outside of the HMO system, PPOs will pay part of the costs if a member receives care from a doctor, hospital, or other provider that is not part of the plan's network.

How Patients Get Care

PPOs offer members the choice of using preferred ("in-network") providers at an established rate of coverage or using non-preferred ("out-of-network") providers with reduced coverage. For example, if you use an in-network doctor, the plan may cover 80–100% of your care, while if you receive the same services from a non-network physician, the plan would cover only 60–70% of the in-network fee schedule for your care. For out-of-network care, you are responsible for paying the other 30–40% of the fee schedule—plus 100% of the amount the doctor charges above the fee schedule.

Insurance Hassles

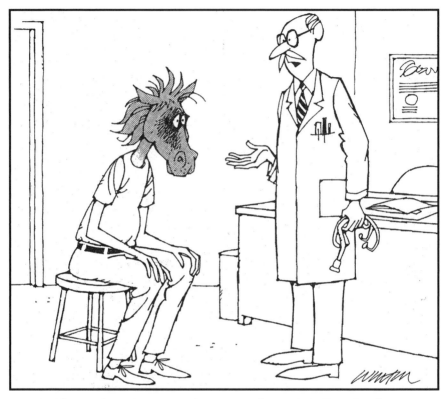

"WHEN YOU SAID YOU'D BEEN TALKING TO YOUR INSURANCE COMPANY UNTIL YOU WERE GETTING HOARSE, I HAD NO IDEA…."

Preferred and non-preferred providers can be used simultaneously. Doctors are usually required to get approval from the plan before sending patients to the hospital and possibly for certain types of special outpatient procedures, but there are few other rules or regulations for how to get care. The plan does not require the member to use a primary-care physician. Usually, patients are not required to pay the full charges up front or submit claim forms for care received from in-network providers. However, they must do so for care received from out-of-network providers.

How Providers Are Paid

PPO providers are usually reimbursed through a discounted fee arrangement. Doctors join the PPO network in exchange for specific fees for each type of service they actually provide. Non-PPO rates for services are usually averaged for each geographic area. Then those average rates are discounted by a specified percentage for the PPO doctors. The doctors agree to the discount because the health plan will generate more traffic for them—marketing on their behalf—by putting them on the "preferred" list.

In-network doctors must agree not to charge patients more than the plan's copay and/or coinsurance amount. Then they bill the health plan for the additional amount—up to the maximum set by the discounted fee schedule. Because the health plan has no contract whatsoever with out-of-network doctors, these doctors are reimbursed by the health plan based either on a percentage of the "usual and customary" rate for that geographic area or on the same fee schedule used for in-network doctors.

The member usually must pay the out-of-network doctor's entire bill, and then submit a claim to the health plan for reimbursement. The health plan then reimburses the patient the discounted "usual and customary" amount, less any deductible and/or coinsurance. The member does not get reimbursed for the percentage of the "usual and customary" charges *not* covered by the health plan—usually 20-30%. Nor does the patient get reimbursed for any amount of the charges over and above the "usual and customary" amount if the doctor charged more than average.

Financial Forces Impacting Your Care

Just like regular, old-fashioned fee-for-service, discounted fee-for-service systems motivate providers to give you as many services as they can justify in order to give themselves as

> Because you don't need a referral from a primary-care doctor to see a specialist, getting care is simpler and more hassle-free in a PPO than in a network-model HMO.

much income as possible. As a result, at least some of the care patients receive may not be necessary.

As mentioned in our discussion of indemnity plans, the fee-for-service payment mechanism also tends to encourage providers to concentrate on illness care over preventive care. In addition to the fact that it may be more interesting, treating illness almost always pays the provider more.

Ease of Getting Care

Because you don't need a referral from a primary-care doctor to see a specialist, getting care is simpler and more hassle-free in a PPO than in a network-model HMO. It is fairly easy to use a PPO as long as you make sure to use in-network providers. Once you go out of the plan's network, the hassles increase for getting claims paid, the costs of care go up, and you must submit claim forms to get reimbursed for the out-of-network care you receive.

Sometimes, patients don't realize they are using an out-of-network doctor. As more doctors drop out of networks, it becomes more frequent that patients keep going to their regular doctor without realizing he or she is no longer in-network. Be sure to check each time you call your doctor to schedule an appointment that he or she is still in-network and plans to continue to be.

A recent survey by *Consumer Reports* of 42,000 readers showed that billing and customer service problems are more common to PPOs than to HMOs.[1] The same survey reported that people with chronic problems had the same levels of satisfaction with HMOs and PPOs, except for people with back pain and arthritis, who preferred PPOs.

Costs

Just like straight fee-for-service in indemnity plans, the discounted fee payment arrangement in PPOs motivates doctors to give patients more services than may be necessary. This fee-for-service payment method is a key reason PPO plans are generally more expensive than HMOs. Doctors often feel justified prescribing extra care—one more test to make sure, etc. But, as stated above, bottom-line medical necessity is often questionable. Because patients usually pay only a small part of the total costs, they have little financial incentive to question the necessity of services prescribed by a PPO doctor or given by a PPO hospital—especially since patients often (erroneously) believe that more care is better care.

> Just like straight fee-for-service in indemnity plans, the discounted fee payment arrangement in PPOs motivates doctors to give patients more services than may be necessary.

Quality

Desiring freedom of choice, those consumers who can afford it often choose PPO plans, and quite a few use out-of-network doctors. Many assume that this gives them the best possible care. However, because the quality of care given by most doctors is very difficult to measure and compare, there is no way to be sure they are providing high-quality care. Even most in-network PPO doctors are not held accountable for quality. While there is a growing movement to measure and compare the care provided by PPOs, few PPOs participate in valid measurement programs.

Pros

Freedom of choice: If there are high-quality providers on the PPO's in-network list, you can use them while getting the most coverage. However, even if the highest-quality providers are not on the list, you can still use them and get some coverage. But don't assume you know who the high-quality providers are. Use medical group and hospital quality comparison surveys to find out for sure.

Cons

It is difficult to measure or compare the quality of care provided by PPO doctors because few quality comparisons are available for PPOs (though some of the participating medical groups and hospitals may participate in quality surveys). Overall costs tend to be higher than for HMOs. The fee-for-service payment method encourages providers to overuse medical care, which can put patients at unnecessary risk. The fee-for-service arrangement also encourages doctors to concentrate on treating disease rather than on ensuring wellness.

Ppos—Summary

Overall Value

• The value of PPO plans varies. The value of a particular PPO plan depends on the total costs to you and the level of quality you can get in that plan compared to your other choices.

• The quality of care in a PPO depends on whether the network is composed of high-quality doctors and hospitals. The total cost depends on the combination of your monthly and per-use costs. Per-use costs depend on whether you use in-network or out-of-network providers. You must use in-network providers to pay the least for each service you receive.

• You may be able to get equal or better quality and satisfaction in a good HMO plan for less overall cost.

• If you do not have a good HMO plan available, use a PPO wisely by making sure to get all appropriate preventive services and by using only the high-quality providers on its list.

Clinical Quality

(–) Few PPOs collect data for quality measurement, so few PPOs are surveyed for quality comparison.

(+) Legitimate quality assessment organizations are now starting to review PPOs for quality of care.

(–) No guarantee of quality. Choose MD and hospital carefully.

Ease of Getting Care

(+) In PPOs there is the convenience of being able to use any doctor you wish. Even if the doctor you want to see is not on the plan's preferred list, you still get some coverage.

(–) You must usually go to multiple locations to get all of your services.

(–) The process for getting authorization for nonemergency inpatient care can be cumbersome in some plans. Check consumer satisfaction ratings of any plan you are considering joining.

(–) Claim forms need to be submitted for out-of-network services to be covered by the plan. Understanding and tracking how claims are paid can be cumbersome and confusing.

Costs
(±) When the amount of coverage and total out-of-pocket costs are considered, PPOs generally fall between HMOs and straight indemnity plans in costs.

20 Epos

*Money is the opposite of the weather. Nobody talks about it,
but everybody does something about it.*
—Rebecca Johnson, in *Vogue*

In This Chapter...
A description of many aspects of EPO plans and a chart
that summarizes them.

Background

Exclusive Provider Organizations (EPOs) were developed
as a variation on HMOs. Usually there is a specified list of
doctors and hospitals that patients must use to receive coverage, which makes EPOs look like HMOs. However, EPOs are
not as tightly regulated by federal and state laws as are HMOs.
This gives them more flexibility in designing the benefits they
cover plus a few other aspects of greater freedom of design
and administration that HMOs do not have. EPO doctors are
usually reimbursed on a discounted fee-for-service arrangement, like PPO in-network physicians, which many doctors
prefer over the "per-head" (capitated) payment arrangements
of many HMOs.

How Patients Get Care

Just as in network-model HMOs, members of EPO plans must
usually specify a primary-care physician (PCP), who autho-
rizes all of that member's care, including referrals to specialists. Also as in HMOs, the specialists to whom the patient is
referred must usually be in the PCP's medical group.

How Providers Are Paid

As mentioned above, EPO doctors are generally paid on a
discounted fee-for-service basis, like PPO doctors. The EPO
doctors must not charge patients more than the plan's copay.

The doctors must then collect the rest of the agreed-upon discounted fee from the health plan.

Financial Forces Impacting Your Care

The health plan is able to control costs through discounted fees, but the same financial incentives that apply to doctors under fee-for-service remain: Do more in order to increase income. Total premium costs for EPOs are generally higher than HMOs, though patient copayments and other out-of-pocket costs related to use of services are often very similar to HMOs.

Ease of Getting Care

Some of the same restrictions apply to getting care in EPOs as do in HMOs. In most EPO plans, you must use only the providers on the plan's list in order to get coverage, and there are usually rules for getting authorizations and referrals for anything beyond a visit to your PCP.

The rare instances in which you might want to challenge your plan's decision about your care can be time-consuming and daunting. Although public perception is that this is truer in HMOs, it is actually just as true in other types of plans when care requires preauthorization. And because HMOs are the most highly regulated of all plans, there is generally more state-level assistance for grievance processes in HMOs than in other types of plans. In other words, you may get more assistance from your state government if you have a problem with an HMO than if you have a problem with an EPO or other type of plan.

Costs

Costs for copayments in EPOs are often about the same as in HMOs—generally lower than in most other types of plans. However, monthly premiums for EPOs are often higher than for HMOs in the same geographic area. Again, think about the financial incentives for doctors: In EPOs, doctors are paid on a discounted fee-for-service basis, which encourages them to prescribe more care than may be clearly needed. Compare that to doctors' financial incentives in HMOs, which encourage doctors to provide all necessary care within a preset budget, with the danger in some cases of skimping on care.

If you personally do not have to pay the full amount of the monthly premium (e.g., if your employer pays part of it), you may prefer the risk of being over-treated to being denied treatment, and thus you may prefer an EPO to an HMO. However, bear in mind the following:

1. Ultimately we all pay for excess healthcare costs. Excess costs increase premiums, and as total healthcare costs increase, the increase is paid for by employers by putting a damper on wage increases, or in other ways that ultimately have a negative impact on employees.

2. Unnecessary care often puts the patient at risk in some way. If, for example, you are prescribed a drug that you don't really need, you may suffer detrimental side effects from that drug. In that case, you and your employer will pay an increase in premium due to the cost of the unnecessary drug, the doctor's time in prescribing it, plus the costs of diagnosing and treating the side effect.

The rare instances in which you might want to challenge your plan's decision about your care can be time-consuming and daunting.

Over-treatment is not necessarily preferable to under-treatment. The best approach is to use a medical group and health plan that is highly rated on quality, so that both your doctor and health plan pay attention to quality issues. Then you must take the additional step of researching what care is best for your situation, and then work with your doctor to make sure that all appropriate—and no inappropriate—care is provided.

Quality

EPO doctors are sometimes, though rarely, required to let the health plan collect information from patient charts in order to measure quality. If the doctor also participates in an HMO, his or her care may be measured through that affiliation, possibly giving consumers some information about the level of quality being provided.

Pros

Costs: The positive aspects of EPOs are primarily financial. Doctors, hospitals, and other providers contract with the health plan and agree to receive lower payments for services in exchange for having patients directed to them. The health plan can, in turn, charge lower premiums for these plans than for PPO or POS plans, which do not restrict members to use only network providers. This lower cost aspect of EPOs holds true as long as the set of benefits on the EPO plan is not substantially richer than a PPO plan. If the benefits are significantly richer than a comparative PPO plan, the total premium costs may be about the same or higher than PPOs.

Cons

Quality: EPO plans are not usually included in the third-party surveys that compare the quality of different health plans.

Therefore, quality assurance mechanisms are not usually emphasized in EPO provider contracts.

Choice: You must use the plan's doctors and hospitals. This can be good or bad, depending on the level of quality of these providers.

EPOs—Summary

Overall Value

• Can be a good value if high-quality MDs and hospitals are on the list and if your other choices are more expensive.

Clinical Quality

(−) No guarantee of quality. Choose MD and hospital carefully.

(−) EPOs generally do not incorporate patient care data collection mechanisms and therefore are not able to measure quality of care.

Ease of Getting Care

(+) You may find more MDs on EPO lists than on HMO lists.

(−) In almost all EPO plans, you will be locked into the EPO list of providers. You must receive all your care from providers on the plan's list in order to have your care covered.

(−) There is generally less state-level assistance for member grievances with EPOs and other types of plans than with HMOs.

Costs

(+) EPOs are generally less expensive than PPOs, POS plans, and indemnity plans.

(−) EPOs tend to be more expensive than HMOs.

---

21 POS Plans

A billion here, a billion there, and pretty soon you're talking about real money. —Everett Dirksen

In This Chapter...
A description of many aspects of POS plans and a chart that summarizes them.

Background

Point of Service (POS) plans were created as another response to consumers' resentment about being locked into HMO physician lists. A number of POS plans began to appear on the market during the late 1980s and early 1990s. These plans are an HMO and a PPO folded into one arrangement, with some advantages and disadvantages of each.

How Patients Get Care

POS plans are usually composed of three "tiers" of choices. The first is the HMO tier, in which the member can choose from a list of HMO-network physicians. The benefits under this tier are usually more generous than under either of the other two tiers, and the copayments are less.

The second tier is composed of a larger network of physicians, hospitals, and other providers. The member can use this tier of PPO providers either *instead of* or *in addition to* the first tier. So, for example, you could see a primary-care physician in the HMO network for all your preventive care and a cardiologist on the PPO list for your high blood pressure problems. In the PPO tier, either the benefits are less generous or the copayments are higher—or both—compared to the HMO tier. For example, the HMO tier may require a $10 office visit copay, while the PPO tier requires a $20 office visit copay.

The third tier allows plan members to use any doctor outside of the HMO or PPO. Let's say you use a PCP on the HMO list for your preventive care, the cardiologist on the PPO list for your high blood pressure care, and your favorite allergist who is not on either the HMO tier or the PPO tier, to help you control your seasonal allergies. Your coverage for using the allergist or any doctor or hospital not on either the HMO or PPO list will be less than on the other two tiers. For example, if you had seen an allergist on the HMO list, your office visit copay might have been $10 (assuming you had gotten the referral from your PCP, if necessary), while if you had seen an allergist on the PPO list your office visit copay might have been $20. Using the out-of-network allergist means you pay maybe 30% of the negotiated fee schedule that would have been paid to the in-network PPO allergist, plus 100% of any amount on top of the negotiated fee amount that your out-of-network allergist charges. So it will cost you a lot more to see the out-of-network doctor, but at least you have some coverage for these visits.

POS plans are usually composed of three "tiers" of choices.

To summarize, members can use providers on any one of the three tiers at any time. Members have the biggest financial incentive to use the HMO tier, somewhat less financial incentive but more choice of providers on the in-network PPO tier, and the least financial incentive but the broadest choice of doctors on the out-of-network tier.

How Providers Are Paid

Providers on the HMO tier are paid just like doctors in a straight HMO plan. Providers in the PPO network are paid just like in any straight PPO plan, as are out-of-network providers.

Financial Forces Impacting Your Care

The same financial incentives apply to each tier of a POS plan, respectively, as apply to a straight HMO (for tier 1) and to a straight PPO (for tiers 2 and 3).

Ease of Getting Care

If you get all your care in the HMO part of the plan (tier 1)—as many POS members do to save money—you will have generally the same experiences in getting care that members of a straight HMO have. How easy it is to get care depends largely on which plan you choose. Find a plan that rates highly in customer satisfaction surveys. Getting care in tiers 2 and 3, including getting claims paid, will be similar to getting care in a regular PPO. One difference may be that, due to the complexity of the POS structure, insurance companies sometimes have a harder time keeping straight which tier you used for a particular service. There may be problems with claims payments or other types of administrative issues as a result.

Costs

The total current premium costs of POS plans are now often about the same as or somewhat higher than those of straight PPO plans. Originally POS plan premiums were lower than PPO plans because insurance companies expected that the lower cost and cost control features of the HMO tier would keep the total costs down. One reason costs are higher than originally projected for POS plans is that it costs the insurance company more to administer this complex type of plan than either a straight HMO or a straight PPO plan.

Employees in some companies are offered a choice between a regular HMO plan and a POS plan. When monthly employee contribution costs are about the same for the HMO and the POS plans, many employees choose the POS plan even if they only use the HMO tier because they then have the option to use the PPO part of the plan at any time. In contrast, if they enroll in the straight HMO, they do not get any coverage when using providers outside the HMO's list. However, if the monthly employee contribution for the POS is much higher than for the HMO, and if the employee is most likely going to use only HMO providers, then it makes more sense to choose the HMO plan.

A similar scenario would apply in companies that offer employees a choice between a regular PPO and a POS plan. If the monthly employee contribution costs are essentially the same for both plans, many employees choose the POS plan because it gives them more options for care.

However, nowadays more employers are making employees pay the difference between the various types of plans offered. In this case, you must weigh out how much the "just in case" choice option is worth to you.

> When you use unconnected providers, the coordination and therefore the quality of your care often suffers.

Quality

Because POS plans are hybrids, containing elements of both HMOs and PPOs, the same quality assessments can be applied to each tier of POS plans as apply to HMO and PPO plans respectively. The only difference is that, because patients are not locked into any one tier, all of their care cannot necessarily be measured. So you may not be able to find any quality assessments comparing POS plans.

Pros

Flexibility: In a POS plan, you have the flexibility to take advantage of lower costs using the HMO network for some care and a greater choice of providers using the PPO tier for other care. However, due to the added costs of using non-network providers, many POS plan members wind up just using the HMO network. Therefore, look carefully at the extra costs you could pay for flexibility that you may never use.

Cons

Quality: When you use unconnected providers, the coordination and therefore the quality of your care often suffers.

Costs: POS plans are generally more expensive than HMO plans. If you must pay the difference in premiums, carefully evaluate the real advantages you are paying for. If you have the option, a high-quality HMO may give you better value.

POS Plans—Summary

Overall Value

• If being locked into an HMO's list of providers really bothers you, this type of plan, if available, may be the best value for you. However, the administrative costs of POS plans tend to be high, so compare costs carefully.

Clinical Quality

(+) The HMO tier of these plans may be a part of a standard HMO plan that is surveyed and rated for quality, in which case you may be able to choose a POS plan and use the HMO tier with assurance of getting a certain level of quality. In addition, you still have the option to use the PPO tiers of the plan whenever you wish, though you will have to choose your PPO-tier MD carefully to get the best quality.

(–) No guarantee of quality in any of the tiers. You must choose your MD and hospital carefully to get high quality.

Ease of Getting Care

(+) Wide choice of providers and types of care: You have the option of getting HMO care, in-network PPO care, or out-of-network care.

(+) Flexibility: You can use care in any of the tiers at any time.

(±) Your experiences in getting care in any of the tiers will be similar to getting care in a health plan that offers only that type of care (HMO or PPO).

Costs

(+) Your total costs for HMO (first-tier) or in-network PPO (second-tier) care can be relatively low, depending on your plan.

(–) Usually more expensive than regular HMOs.

22 Consumer-Directed and VIP Plans

If opportunity doesn't knock, build a door.
—Milton Berle

In This Chapter...
- A description of many aspects of "consumer-directed" plans.
- A description of VIP plans.

"Consumer-Directed" Plans

Healthcare costs are rising at an alarming rate, faster than many employers can absorb. Costs of employer-sponsored health benefits increased an average of 13.9% between the Springs of 2002 and 2003—making it the highest premium increase since 1990.[1] Employee benefits costs, primarily driven by healthcare benefits, are rising 300% faster than average wages.[2] At this rate, healthcare benefits costs will double in a little more than seven years. In the 1960s, employees shared roughly one-half of health benefits costs with employers. By 1999 employees' average share of costs had dropped to 17%.[3] Something has to give.

This situation has led many employers to be very interested in a new type of health plan, called a "consumer-driven" or "consumer-directed" plan. The goal of these plans is to make consumers responsible for more of the total healthcare bill, forcing consumers to purchase only the healthcare services they need. When we pay only a relatively small portion of the bill, we don't tend to pay keen attention to the full cost of the services we use. We tend to accept whatever our doctors prescribe for us. We don't question whether it is really necessary. By putting more of the payment responsibility on our shoulders, employers hope that employees will become more responsible about how we use healthcare. The theory is that we will question the necessity of every healthcare service we must now pay for. As you will see below, the new plans have pros and cons for consumers, and they may or may not achieve the desired goal.

How the Plans Are Designed

A typical consumer-driven plan would make each employee responsible for the first $1,500 of his or her healthcare costs each year. The amount varies by plan, but the idea is that it is a much bigger chunk of our initial annual expenses than we are used to handling. Don't panic quite yet. To help offset this $1,500 responsibility, the employer would (in most of these proposed plans) put aside a substantial amount of money annually for each employee, say $1,000, in a special account that the employee can use for any healthcare expenses of his or her choice. After the employee spends the $1,000 put aside by the employer, the employee would be responsible to pay the next $500 out-of-pocket before the health plan would start its coverage. In essence, the health plan has a very high deductible.

> Roughly 10% of the population is responsible for roughly 80% of total healthcare costs.

Another key feature of these arrangements is that if the employee does not use the full $1,000 that year, the remainder gets rolled over for use in the next or following years, with the standard $1,000 added each year. The idea is that employees would be encouraged to save as much of the $1,000 each year as possible, so as to have it available if they need it in following years. Remember, the specific dollar amounts in this illustration are just an example. The amount of the deductible as well as the amount funded by the employer will vary.

How These Plans Are Offered

Of the few employers who have implemented consumer-driven plans, many have offered them as an option alongside other traditional types of coverage, like HMOs and PPOs. Employees therefore have a choice about participating in the new plan. Usually, the monthly contribution for employees who choose the new plan is substantially less than that for the other plans offered.

Cost Control Is in Our Best Interests

Keep in mind that, although our employers have been paying directly for a large portion of the total health insurance bill, we have paid indirectly for these costs through loss of potential wages, loss of jobs, or in some other way. And there is strong evidence that 30% of healthcare is wasted in the form of misuse, overuse, or underuse.[4] So any new way to effectively control costs is generally in our best interests. However, here are a few cautionary notes about the new consumer-directed plans:

- Roughly 10% of the population is responsible for roughly 80% of total healthcare costs. These are the sickest among us. The rest of us who are healthier are responsible for only about 20% of the total costs. It is the upper-end, high-dollar care for the very sick that needs to be managed most.

  Having employees manage the first $1,500 of their annual expenses may put only a very small dent in the total costs of an employer's health benefits bill. To really have an impact on total healthcare costs, some significant cost-control mechanism needs to be built into the plan that takes over after the initial deductible has been met. Excellent disease management programs, including one-on-one health coaching, should be included in these plans.

- There is some evidence from the first few employers who have implemented these plans that the participating employees have reduced the overall costs of care, though only slightly, especially in the use of prescription drugs. More generics were substituted for brand-name drugs, for example, and the overall use of drugs decreased. If this is the only significant change in purchasing patterns the new plans bring about, it will not make a big enough difference in the long run.

- If employees have a choice of health plans, these new plans may tend to first attract the younger, healthier employees who don't use much healthcare. These employees will tend to see the new options as a low-cost yet fairly low-risk way to get healthcare coverage. This will tend to leave the older and sicker employees (or those with dependents who need a lot of care) in the traditional HMO and PPO plans.

  Having all the sicker employees and dependents in the traditional plans, without the lower-cost, younger employees in these plans to balance the risk and spread the cost, will drive up the average costs of these traditional plans over time. This will make the traditional plans increasingly unaffordable, especially to the younger employees who are just getting started on the salary/wage ladder as well as for those who are in the lower-wage job categories. The higher and higher costs of the traditional plans could eventually force all employees into the new plan because no one will be able to afford the traditional plans. It is too soon to tell if this would be a good or a bad result.

- Those who use a lot of healthcare services—the sickest employees and dependents—will have less incentive to manage the first $1,500 of their care (or whatever the amount of the full deductible on any particular consumer-driven plan) because they will spend that amount very quickly each year.

- Consumer-directed plan participants may be tempted to save money by skimping on preventive care. This, of course, will increase not only costs but more importantly it will increase disability in the long term. Therefore consumer-directed plans should be designed to encourage use of preventive care. This can be accomplished, for example, if employers provide 100% coverage for appropriate preventive services all year every year for every employee and dependent, on top of providing the $1,000 (or whatever amount) in the special fund.

- Consumers also may avoid appropriate care when an illness is in its early stages if the patient has not yet spent the full deductible and reached the higher level of coverage. For example, diabetics need to have regular contact with their doctors and get all the care necessary to keep their blood glucose levels under control. Skimping on this type of care would be a negative result of a consumer-directed plan, yet so far there are few financial mechanisms in these types of plans to discourage this type of skimping on the part of consumers who have not yet met their annual deductible.

- Consumer-driven plan participants may focus only on the cost of the services they want to purchase, disregarding quality comparisons. To get better value for their healthcare dollars, all consumers need better education about quality of care and how the healthcare system works. However, this is especially true for employees who choose to participate in the new consumer-driven plans. Employers who implement these new plans should be aware of this and should provide assistance and/or direction to employees to get this education and encouragement.

Will Your Employer Offer a Consumer-Directed Plan?

Very few employers have offered these new plans to date, and these have done so only very recently. However, many employers are interested in consumer-directed plans. Most employers are cautiously waiting to see the first results of the plans now in place. Preliminary results show a trend in the new plans toward lower overall costs without any apparent serious adverse affects, so it is likely that we will begin to see more and more employers offering these new plans to their employees.

The first implementers were very large employers, and it is other very large employers who are most likely to be next, followed by mid-size employers. One recent survey report predicted that the number of large employers offering a consumer-directed type of plan will quadruple in 2003 to 16%.[5] As this book goes to press, it is too early to confirm the accuracy of this prediction, but it is clear that implementation of consumer-directed plans is growing. Because small employers have the biggest challenges related to cost increases, even they may start implementing these plans soon, but only time will tell the full story.

> Healthcare costs are rising at an alarming rate, faster than many employers can absorb.

VIP Plans

Some doctors, frustrated with the huge amount of administrative hassle and the challenges to their authority in making treatment decisions for patients, are now refusing to accept payment directly through insurance. Instead, they are setting up "boutique" practices in which patients pay a retainer fee. These retainer fees range between $900 and $20,000 per year.[6]

In exchange for this fee, the patient receives better access to the doctor and more personalized care than the doctor is able to offer otherwise. The patient is entirely responsible for getting reimbursement from his or her insurance company, if possible. The doctor usually has fewer patients overall but receives the same or possibly a better income than when being a preferred provider for multiple insurance companies.

For patients who can afford the high retainer fees, these arrangements may be a nice solution to getting more attention from their doctor. One major catch in these arrangements, though, is that most of us can't afford the high retainer fees. Another major problem is that the doctor may or may not be providing the best quality medical care. Again, please remember that more attention and better "beside manner" are not the same as technical quality of care.

PART VI
OTHER HELPFUL INFORMATION

Chapter 23
Balancing Cost and Quality

Chapter 24
The Path Less Traveled: Alternative Medicine

Chapter 25
It's No Easier for the Doctors

Chapter 26
You *Can* Make a Difference in Your Healthcare

These final chapters are filled with important information on a variety of topics, all indirectly related to the purpose of this book: helping you to find the best quality in medical care.

The last chapter, Chapter 26, summarizes all the recommendations I have given you throughout the book and gives a bit of final advice.

23 Balancing Cost and Quality

We learn the rope of life by untying its knots.
—Jean Toomer

In This Chapter...
- Healthcare costs are rising at an alarming rate.
- YOU pay for most of these cost increases, in ways you may not realize.
- Good healthcare is not cheap.
- An estimated 30% of all U.S. healthcare is wasteful.
- Factors contributing to increasing costs.

Skyrocketing Costs

As mentioned in Chapter 22, U.S. healthcare costs have been increasing at double-digit rates each year since the late 1990s. Between the Springs of 2002 and 2003, monthly premiums for employer-sponsored health insurance rose 13.9%.[1] At this rate, our healthcare will double in cost within eight years.

At the time this book went to print, the average annual HMO health insurance premiums across the nation had risen to $3,154 for single coverage and $8,514 for family coverage. For PPO coverage, average annual premiums were $3,505 for single coverage and $9,317 for family coverage. Premiums increased substantially faster than overall inflation (2.2%) and wage gains for non-supervisory workers (3.1%).[2]

Of the total premium costs, employees paid on average only $502 annually for single HMO coverage and $2,145 for family coverage. For PPO coverage, employees paid $527 on average annually for single coverage and $2,515 for family coverage.[3] Also mentioned in Chapter 22, in the 1960s, employees shared roughly one-half of health benefits costs with employers. By 1999 employees' average share of costs had dropped to 17%. However, according to the U.S. Bureau of Labor Statistics, there has been a 75% average increase in premiums paid by

Medical Devices Keep Advancing

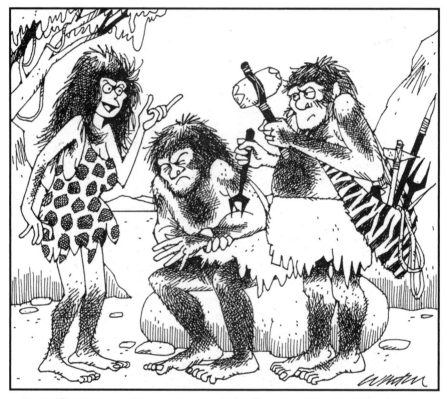

"YOUR NEW MEDICAL DEVICES ARE PRETTY IMPRESSIVE, DOC, BUT I BET THEY'LL BE ENVIRONMENTAL CLUTTER FOR EONS."

employees for their share of health coverage over the past decade, obviously significantly outpacing wages or inflation.[4]

So, on average, consumers who get health benefits through employers are paying a much smaller portion of the overall healthcare bill now than folks did in the 1960s. However, that portion had dipped to its lowest in 1999. Since then, consumers' portion of the cost has been increasing substantially. Since most of us only see what has been happening recently, many people are strongly objecting to the recent increases in their share of costs. At the same time, they are unable to see that part of the cause of increasing costs is consumers' unawareness of costs. In fact, consumers' direct out-of-pocket healthcare expenses are still less than 20% of the total bill. Being unaware of the huge total costs, we tend to be too careless about how we spend. We rarely ask our doctors if a test is really necessary, for example, because we don't have to pay the whole cost. And we tend to just trust our doctor to prescribe only what is necessary. Sometimes that is a big mistake!

Healthcare represents 14% of the U.S. gross domestic product (GDP), and that percentage continues to grow. Total U.S. healthcare expenditures are projected to increase from $1.31 trillion in 2000 to $2.6 trillion in 2010, representing 16% of GDP.[5]

To give you an idea of just how much healthcare costs have increased compared to other goods and services we use every day, if food had increased in cost as much as healthcare since the 1930s, a dozen eggs would cost about $45 today![6] Yes, it's that bad.

Most employers pay more every year to provide their employees with healthcare benefits. Many employers pass some of these increases on to employees by taking higher monthly contributions out of their paychecks, or by increasing copayments and coinsurance. Many large and mid-size employers are not yet passing on the entire annual increase in healthcare costs to employees (at least not directly; read on for the real story). But many small and mid-size employers can no longer afford to absorb the increases. The number of employed people who no longer have healthcare benefits is increasing, as are the number of people who do not have health insurance coverage of any kind.

> The number of employed people who no longer have healthcare benefits is increasing, as are the number of people who do not have health insurance coverage of any kind.

You Probably Pay More Than You Know

Though employees with healthcare benefits are being asked to pay more and more for their care and coverage, few realize

263

how much their employers spend for their coverage on their behalf. The figures above will give you a clue. Most employees assume the employer easily absorbs these costs, minus the employees' monthly contributions, as a cost of doing business. But think about it. If a business's revenues increase 2% per year, for example, the business can absorb increased costs of doing business at about that same rate of increase, 2%. If any particular cost of doing business rises much faster than average revenues—as healthcare costs have been doing for some time—those extra costs must come out of some other pot.

The U.S. healthcare system is riddled with tremendous waste and unnecessary costs.

The fact is that the "other pot" employers dip into is often salaries and wages. You may not be paying the entire amount of healthcare cost increases directly, but you are probably paying through curbed wage increases—or even the loss of your job as employers downsize to decrease overall costs. So the cost of healthcare is something that should interest you greatly and that you should understand well.

The full costs of healthcare have been shielded from consumers far too long. As a result, many consumers are less than fully sensitive to the cost/coverage/quality trade-offs that should be at the heart of every decision about healthcare coverage and services. If you think you don't pay the full costs of healthcare, think again.

Some Good News

Americans have been getting healthier, at least in part, because of our healthcare. In 1980, life expectancy in the U.S. was 73.7 years. By 1996, it had increased to 76.1 years, and it continues to improve. Between 1980 and 1996, death rates from heart disease decreased by 9% and from cancer by 4%. Though many other factors have also contributed to improvements in our longevity and quality of life over the past century, such as safer and less physically punishing jobs, it is certainly true that constant improvements in medical care have contributed and continue to contribute to our well-being. None of us would seriously consider stopping improvements in medicine, even though they are expensive.

The Waste Factor

Yes, healthcare improvements are expensive, but let's not add to the problem by being wasteful! Many healthcare industry insiders have known for some time that the U.S. healthcare system is riddled with tremendous waste and unnecessary costs, but until very recently, no one could quantify the problem. Then in June 2002, the Midwest Business Group on Health, a Chicago-based coalition of large employers, reported the results of a carefully designed research project they had taken on to get some answers.[7] The study shows that a whopping 30% of costs result directly from administrative inefficiencies and misuse (overuse, underuse of preventive care, and wrong use) of medical services. The study also addresses indirect costs, such as reduced employee productivity due to unnecessary illness, which wasn't even included in the 30% waste figure. The real cost of the waste in the system is therefore even higher than 30%.

The report points to employers as partly to blame for these unjustified costs. By using "transaction-based" rather than "outcomes-based" payment structures, employers have contributed to the problem. (In a transaction-based system, doctors and other providers are paid for each service rendered; in an outcomes-based system, providers would only be paid if your health improves as a result of their care.) Transaction-based payment encourages doctors, hospitals, and other care providers to promote the use of healthcare services even if they don't improve health. Additionally, it discourages providers from improving quality.

Employers have further added to the problem by making health-plan contracting decisions based on price alone, without considering the quality-of-care performance history of the plan or the provider. And they rarely inform or educate employees about healthcare quality issues.

But the report also shows that consumers share the blame. As stated before, consumers have not had much incentive to care about overall costs. In addition, as patients we hold firmly to the belief that we should get as much medical care as we need, regardless of costs. I, too, believe that we all deserve all the healthcare we need, whether or not we can individually afford it, but the problem is that we've been poorly educated about what we need. We as consumers have not been told about the huge gaps in quality in our care, or about the massive waste in dollars—not to mention health—associated with that poor quality.

Irony #1

Americans pay more for healthcare than any other country in the world. Yet…generally, we do not get good value for our money. We are not the healthiest nation in the world, and we get far fewer healthcare services for our money per person than in other countries that spend much less on healthcare per person.[8]

Factors That Are Increasing Costs

Some causes of increasing healthcare costs may be justified. Some are not. Here are some of the factors that are contributing to the steep increases in healthcare costs today.

Declining Use of Managed Care

Many consumers flocked to join HMOs in the 1980s and 1990s, attracted by the lower out-of-pocket costs of these plans. But after experiencing frustrations in getting care in many HMOs, some consumers have been opting out of HMOs, mostly to join PPOs instead, because PPOs manage care much less than HMOs do. Unfortunately, this is like throwing the baby out with the bathwater. Because people associate the term "HMO" with poor quality, those HMOs that emphasize high quality and don't frustrate members are getting the same bad rap as the lower-quality HMOs. And many consumers are giving up on HMOs because the reasons for some of the "management" of care have not been explained well.

> Obesity increases risk for Type 2 diabetes, heart disease, stroke, and certain cancers and in the U.S. costs $93 billion in annual medical expenses.

New Equipment and Procedures

Developing new, more-effective medical equipment and procedures is expensive. Providers recover their investments in new diagnostic and therapeutic tools by raising prices for the consumer. Sometimes these new developments replace therapies that were even more costly, thus yielding net savings. Other times they offer more effective or less risky therapy than previous methods. New laser surgery techniques, for example, have made it possible to perform extensive internal surgery with little more than minor incisions. Thus, patients need to spend less time recovering in high-cost hospital settings.

Increasing Costs of Medical Malpractice Insurance

For a variety of reasons, physicians and other providers must now pay more than ever to protect themselves from the potential impact of lawsuits.

An Aging Population

Adults older than 65 use an average of three times as many healthcare services as those under 65. The first wave of baby boomers will turn 65 in 2011. Bottom line, there's not much we can do about the increasing average age of our population. However, as individuals we can control the costs of our own healthcare—and improve our chances of being healthy—by taking prevention seriously.

The Fattening of America

Many unhealthy behaviors contribute to developing expensive illnesses. The costs of care associated with being overweight or obese are significant. Obesity increases risk for Type 2 diabetes, heart disease, stroke, and certain cancers and in the U.S. costs $93 billion in annual medical expenses. About half of these costs are picked up by the government. That leaves quite a chunk paid for by private insurance, mostly employer-paid. This is comparable to the annual medical bill for smoking, and it does not include indirect costs such as lost work time associated with obesity-related illness.[9]

More Use of Services

Some consumers take advantage of the low out-of-pocket cost of doctor office visits offered by many health plans. And, when patients pay only $10 or $20 to see a doctor, they tend to think of medical care as relatively inexpensive. They don't see the real costs or the impact of all their visits on the overall costs of care. In fact, as mentioned earlier, most of us don't have any way of knowing the full costs of our care. No wonder statistics show an increasing use of services, especially in situations where out-of-pocket costs are low.

Labor and Related Costs

Today, there is a shortage of certain types of medical personnel, nurses in particular. As happens in such situations, those who are in short supply can demand and get higher wages. Some hospitals have found that they have cut back too far on their number of nurses, and, as a result, patient care is suffering. Thus, nurse staffing is now on an upswing in order to improve quality of care in hospitals.

Also, doctors and hospitals in some parts of the country, especially on the West Coast, are demanding higher reimbursement rates from health plans after years of having their reimbursement levels ratcheted down by managed care plans.

Inefficiencies in our healthcare systems also cause higher labor costs. When an ineffective treatment doesn't work, additional care is needed, and the overall cost of care is more. Also, when care is poorly coordinated, unnecessary effort (and therefore cost) goes into providing that care.

When increased labor costs improve efficiency and/or patient outcomes, the costs are justified. When the cost of labor increases and all we are accomplishing is maintaining or augmenting the inefficiencies inherent in our current systems, patients don't benefit, and the costs are unwarranted.

> Before designing and passing new legislation, consumers and legislators need to better understand the healthcare system and its problems.

Medical Labor Shortages

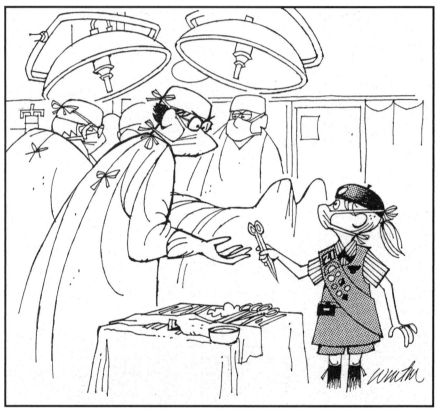

"I KNOW THERE'S A NURSING SHORTAGE,
BUT THIS IS RIDICULOUS."

Doctors, nurses, and other caregivers deserve to be paid well; that is not disputed. We do, however, need to focus on making our healthcare systems more efficient and effective in doing what they are supposed to do—improving people's health.

New Government Mandates

The biggest result of the consumer backlash against healthcare is a frenzy of healthcare-related proposed legislation, some of which will become law. Legislators, desperate to respond to multiple consumer complaints about healthcare, tackle the problems one at a time.

Failing to take a broad view of healthcare issues, legislators have passed regulations that resolve some problems for specific groups but that often neglect the big picture. Creating laws that address only one aspect of the problem can create additional problems. Before designing and passing new legislation, consumers and legislators need to better understand the healthcare system and its problems. That's the only way the system as a whole can improve.

For example, overall costs are going to increase somewhat as a result of patient privacy regulations currently being implemented. All health plans, health insurance carriers, and employers who offer employee health benefits are being required to change the way they track patient care information. Time will tell whether patient privacy legislation actually results in the intended goal and whether the results justify its costs.

New mandates governing healthcare benefits or procedures can create significant administrative and other indirect costs. Legislators need to consider all side effects of potential legislation before making laws.

Increasing Costs of Prescription Drugs

Several important issues affect the prices of prescription drugs. Drug patents, advertising costs, consumer demand for "new and improved" drugs, and low consumer copays all create higher costs for prescription drugs.

When drug manufacturers obtain patents for new drugs, they prevent competitors from making "generic" equivalents for a period of 17 years. During this time, patent holders can charge whatever price they wish for their drugs. This monopoly plays a big part in keeping the costs of many prescription drugs high.

Generic drugs have exactly the same essential chemical components as the original brand-name drug, are just as effective in most cases, and cost much less. Prescribing a brand-name drug is justified in those instances where equivalent generics are not available or where something about the generic does not work for the patient (for example, if the patient has a reaction to the different dye used in the coating of the generic pill). Otherwise, especially given our healthcare-cost crisis, prescribing a brand-name drug when a generic is available is not appropriate.

Expensive furniture in the waiting room or an office in an expensive neighborhood does not mean a physician provides high-quality care.

The ban on drug advertising was lifted in the late 1990s, and drug companies now spend billions on direct-to-consumer advertising, adding to their already high overhead. The new "retail" advertising has resulted in such huge increases in sales that the drug companies will continue to pour vast amounts of money in that direction, increasing the price of the drugs to cover their advertising costs.

And such advertisements are having their effect. Without providing any actual proof, the drug companies have succeeded in convincing hundreds of thousands of consumers—as well as many doctors—that their new brand-name drugs are better than less-expensive and equally effective generics. Consumers are now requesting the advertised drugs by name, some of which may not be appropriate for their specific conditions. But many patients insist on the brand drug they've seen advertised, fully believing that particular drug to be better. Demands from their patients as well as pressure from and incentives offered by drug company sales representatives influence many doctors to prescribe the more-expensive drug.

The same is true of new drugs being introduced. Drug companies are reaping massive profits from sales of new drugs. Customer demand (resulting from advertising) and pressure from drug sales reps also influence doctors to prescribe these newer drugs, even though they may be no better than their older counterparts. Nothing in the FDA's drug approval process requires a new drug to be safer or more effective than another drug already available, though many consumers assume newly approved drugs must be better. The FDA approval process only requires that the drug be safe and do what it is claimed to do.

Drug manufacturers want to get top prices for their products. Keeping "new and improved" products in front of the consumer allows them to create demand for their new branded drug rather than allowing generic equivalents or just-as-effective older formulations to compete with them. As reported by ABC-TV's Peter Jennings in "Bitter Medicine," a 2002 television report on the drug companies' unwarranted hold on the American public, the drug industry is clearly motivated more by profit than by public health. Drug companies argue that they must charge the current high prices to fund ongoing research—but this does not wash. Drug company profits after deducting research costs have grown enormously.

Consumers with health insurance rarely pay the full cost of expensive new drugs. They usually pay a copayment that is only a small portion of the full cost. The patient's prescription drug plan covers the difference. So the patient receives the "benefit" of the expensive drug—whether high, minimal, or nonexistent—and the rest of us subsidize the full cost by paying increasingly more expensive health-plan premiums.

High-quality healthcare reduces human suffering and disability.

As a consumer, I am willing to help pay the increase in cost of prescription drugs if 1) research yields a wonderfully effective new drug that produces significant health improvements, and 2) that drug is shown to be the most cost-effective treatment. After all, I want to have access to high-gain therapies when I need them. I also don't mind helping to cover research and development costs that yield new drugs to replace invasive surgeries or other higher-risk treatments. However, when new drugs do not result in significant health improvements, their higher costs—especially costs related to massive consumer advertising—are not justified, and I am not happy about paying for them. Nor am I happy knowing that so many people waste money on drugs that have less-expensive, equally effective counterparts.

Cost Doesn't Equal Quality

A prevalent healthcare myth mentioned earlier in this book is that more expensive care is clearly "better" care. Thus, consumers who can afford it tend to choose the doctors and hospitals with the highest rates. Because we have been shielded from information about what high-quality healthcare really is and who is providing it, many consumers just assume that higher cost equals higher quality in healthcare. This myth has led to very poor health results in many instances.

Expensive furniture in the waiting room or an office in an expensive neighborhood does not mean a physician provides high-quality care. In fact, some at the upper end of the fee scale practice solo or in small groups in exclusive neighborhoods or in expensive areas of big cities. *None of these high-overhead situations automatically equates to higher quality.* Unfortunately, hundreds of doctors and many hospitals around the country capitalize on this consumer misconception, charging higher prices and projecting an unearned image of higher quality.

Irony #2

"Exclusive" physicians who charge higher fees may not be able to provide the best care, because they may not participate in a good integrated healthcare system.

When a doctor has done the work to legitimately claim top specialty status and provides the best care available, he or she is justified in charging more than average. But when a doctor charges more than average yet produces patient outcomes no better than those of less-expensive providers, the higher fees are unwarranted. Unjustified higher costs are especially unwarranted if the rest of us have to pay for them through higher health-plan premiums.

Irony #3

Some of the highest-quality providers improve patients' health while keeping their overall costs lower than their competitors'.

The Cost/Quality Trade-Off

Development of new drugs, medical equipment, surgical techniques, and other treatments continues to add to the total costs of healthcare—as does the increasing cost of labor and preventive care. In some instances, these improvements replace more expensive treatments, thus lowering costs overall. In other cases, the total cost of care increases, but health outcomes also improve. But, in still other instances, new, more expensive treatments replace old treatments, new drugs replace old ones, and other costs are added to healthcare without improving people's health. These are the increases in costs we want to prevent, because they provide no additional benefit for the consumer.

Most of our current healthcare systems inadequately review the cost-effectiveness of new treatment methods, new drugs, and other cost-increasing changes. The best you as a consumer can do is to ask your doctor about the costs of any proposed treatments compared to their benefits, and do independent research, using legitimate sources of data.

Getting the Most Bang for Your Buck

Good healthcare systems effectively review new drugs, treatments, and technologies, and then use only the best. They avoid overuse, underuse, and misuse of healthcare services, providing the right care at the right time. They also keep administrative costs to a minimum.

To figure out where to direct your healthcare dollars for the best value, look for innovative, forward-looking providers who maintain below-average cost increases while achieving the highest results in quality surveys. Check to make sure that they also incorporate the following important factors in their care:

- **Prevention:** Do they provide all appropriate preventive screening and treatment at the appropriate time, based on the patient's age, gender, family history, lifestyle, etc.?

- **Low-cost prescriptions:** Do participating providers prescribe the most effective drug with the fewest side effects? Where there are drugs with equivalent efficacy, do they choose the lowest-cost option?

- **Evidence-based medicine:** Do they use scientifically proven diagnostic and treatment techniques to determine the right diagnosis and treatment the first time?

- **Coordinated care:** Do they coordinate care at the right time and in the most effective way to provide all of the ancillary and other services necessary for the best outcome?

Even when it is expensive, the highest-quality care is often less expensive than poorer-quality care, because it avoids providing one unproven treatment after another until some cure is found, and it avoids repeating care, such as when tests and procedures already completed by one doctor are repeated by another. High-quality healthcare reduces human suffering and disability. It also improves the productivity of those consumers who are still in the workforce and allows them to remain productive longer. As I have stated earlier, much disability in this country could be prevented if patients received quality care, including appropriate preventive screening and treatment. The high cost of poor quality includes impairment to quality of life.

24 The Path Less Traveled: Alternative Medicine

I took the road less traveled by, and that has made all the difference.
—Robert Frost

In This Chapter...
- A great many of us now use alternative care.
- Beware of potential problems.
- Some types of alternative care are likely to be both safe and effective.

Many of us, frustrated with conventional medical care, have turned to "complementary or alternative medicine" (CAM) for at least some of our care. In fact, according to a recent *Newsweek* article,[1] U.S. consumers "make more visits to non-conventional healers (some 600 million a year) than we do to MDs." We spend more of our own money on these visits, too—an estimated $30 billion a year! CAM includes all types of alternative therapies, including acupuncture, chiropractic, and a host of other less well-known treatments.

Unfortunately, none of these alternative therapies has undergone rigorous testing to prove either its effectiveness or safety. A few, such as acupuncture and chiropractic, appear to be effective for certain specific conditions. But other alternative approaches have shown no signs of being truly effective.

The shockingly large amount of money being spent on CAM has motivated traditional medicine to undertake testing of the most popular alternative therapies. Large-scale, rigorous studies are currently underway. As specific alternative approaches are proven effective for particular medical problems, we can look forward to seeing them covered in our health plans.

Why People Turn to Alternatives

Why the overwhelming interest in alternative medicine? The *Newsweek* article referenced above sheds some light. It cites "a longing to be cared for" as people's primary motivation for turning to alternative practitioners. People desire the touch and caring of a healer at least as much as they do actual relief of their symptoms.

We've all experienced the impersonal attitude of conventional medicine, which tends to view us as collections of body parts rather than as human beings. A great many of us have found relief in the more personal and holistic approach of alternative practitioners. These professionals are more likely to treat you as a whole person—one whose mind, body, emotions, and spirit all interact as part of your larger health picture. Some conventional doctors are now beginning to incorporate a more holistic viewpoint and more personal interactions into their practices. Seek out those who do.

As specific alternative approaches are proven effective for particular medical problems, we can look forward to seeing them covered in our health plans.

Complementary Care

You may also wish to use alternative therapies in combination with your traditional care. A small but growing number of conventionally trained physicians promote this "complementary care" approach, especially for patients who aren't responding well to conventional therapies. You may find a health plan that covers massage therapy, for example, for patients who have tried all reasonable conventional treatments for low-back pain.

Ideally, we would have much clearer knowledge about which alternative and conventional therapies work well together. Over time, we will get there. In the meantime, willing therapists and patients continue to experiment on a case-by-case basis.

When Considering the Alternative Approach...

In addition to safety and effectiveness, here are some things to think about when considering complementary and alternative therapies:

• Neither conventional nor alternative medicine can provide a quick fix. Your best results will come from preventing the ailment in the first place. If it's too late for that, you need to take a hard look at your lifestyle choices and any aspects of your emotional/spiritual approach to life that may be contributing to the problem. Only you can address that part of the cause and the solution.

• Be careful with herbal supplements or other alternative medications, as some are suspected to be unsafe, especially in combination with certain prescription drugs. And be sure to do your homework before replacing prescription drugs that are known to be effective with unproven and possibly totally ineffective herbs or other alternative substances. At a minimum, let your doctor know in detail the names and dosages of any herbal or other alternative substances you are taking. That way your doctor can avoid prescribing a drug suspected to interact adversely with the substance.

• As in conventional medicine, you'll get the best results by working in partnership with your alternative provider, rather than simply turning over all responsibility for your health to him or her.

Likely Safe and Effective[2]

If your traditional care isn't helping as much as you'd like, you may wish to look into the following alternative or complementary therapies. The National Institutes of Health (NIH) deemed these "likely safe and effective":

> Your best results will come from preventing the ailment in the first place.

• **Acupuncture:** for dental pain and for nausea from chemotherapy.

• **Biofeedback:** for musculoskeletal pain, such as temporomandibular joint disorder (TMJ), a dysfunction of the jaw that causes debilitating pain.

• **Chiropractic:** for acute low-back and neck pain, headaches, and sports injuries.

• **Hypnosis:** for reducing the pain and anxiety of minimally invasive medical procedures as well as for chronic pain, severe burns, and disorders worsened by stress, such as irritable bowel syndrome and eczema.

• **Massage:** for low-back pain.

Spirituality in Healing

Though scientific studies cannot prove it, many people recognize a connection between health and spirituality. There is little doubt that our attitudes, beliefs, and outlook on life have an impact on our health and that positive attitudes in some way help heal even serious illnesses. Some people believe in a connection to a divine essence as the basis for this healing phenomenon. Some believe so strongly in this approach that they rely on prayer exclusively for healing. Others do not rely on prayer or spirituality exclusively but believe in the importance of spirituality in conjunction with medical care.

This book's primary focus is on the scientific approach to medical care. However, even the best of science and modern medicine have many gaps in their ability to prevent and cure illness. I believe that feeling connected to and in harmony with the larger universe, or what I think of as the divine, is necessary to my own mental, spiritual, and physical health. Since the power of spirituality cannot be proven, and something that could be called spirituality obviously has some connection to health, every person should determine how spirituality will be part of his or her health journey.

If you think about the value of spirituality, you may decide to make it a greater part of your quest for good health.

25 It's No Easier for the Doctors

It's hard for a physician to do the right thing in the wrong system.
—Anonymous

In This Chapter...
- Most doctors are not happy with current U.S. healthcare.
- Why doctors find the existing system so difficult.
- How state-of-the-art electronic systems could help (and why doctors avoid them).

We often think of doctors as extremely powerful, but they too are stuck in a system that is in transition and that often doesn't work very well. Surveys reveal that doctors as a group are more frustrated with their profession now than at any other time in modern history.

Doctors are having a hard time adjusting to rapid industry changes. Many are not sure anymore what the "right thing" is, and most of those who see where they need to go cannot find an easy way to make the transition. Many doctors lament that medical care cannot be like it used to be. In this way, they feel much the same as many consumers.

Most doctors went into medicine because they wanted to help people. Many also wanted the income, social respect, power, and independence that characterize the profession, but few would have undertaken the years of intense training without a strong dedication to serving patients. Now, many find themselves unable to serve patients as well as they would like, and at the same time they aren't getting the money, prestige, or power doctors once received. Their independent work styles are also threatened. All in all, for most American doctors the picture is no longer very rosy.

The following story gives us a glimpse into the plight of many of today's healthcare professionals. Though the details of the story do not apply across the board, most doctors are

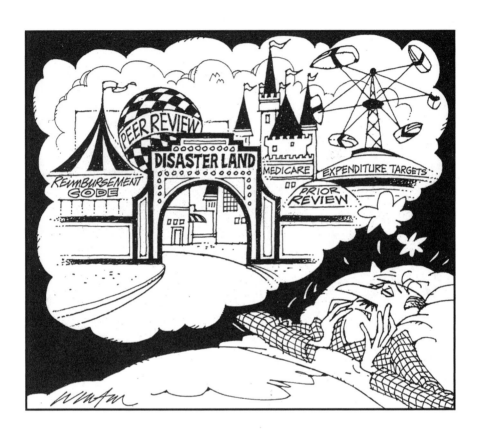

experiencing some aspect of what the physician in the story is going through.

One Physician's Perspective

A 40-something urban doctor who's been practicing for 15 years has become disillusioned about the healthcare system. He works 12 hours a day, takes no vacations, keeps his overheard as low as possible for an independent practitioner, and has trouble paying his taxes.

"Most of my peers are giving up and going to work for the larger HMOs," he says. "There's no security or even much money in being an independent general practitioner, given the huge amounts of paperwork required by the insurers. Why should we work this hard for so little? Face it, the system has failed!"

As a last resort, this doctor is looking into setting himself up with a small number of affluent patients who essentially put him on a retainer—much like lawyers are on retainers—so they have access to him anytime they want to see or consult with him. "This won't make much difference in the larger scope of things," he says, "but it will provide me with a decent income for serving my patients well and not working myself so hard."[1] However, at the prices this doctor and others are proposing to charge for this type of service, most of us can't afford it.

Not only can most people not afford this type of healthcare, but other problems arise with this arrangement, too. We would get more time with our doctor, and our doctor might have increased energy and time for a more caring and humane approach to healing. However, the arrangement would probably not get us the best medical care unless the doctor is part of an integrated support system—which this one is not. And few of us want to hassle with an insurance company on our own without some billing assistance from our doctor's office.

This doctor is caught in a transition period in American medicine. Doctors trying to go it alone may be doomed to fail, as were cottage industries during the industrial revolution. Modern medicine requires a high level of coordination among all types of providers of healthcare, including multiple physician specialties,

Doctors are having a hard time adjusting to rapid industry changes.

Doctors Under Stress

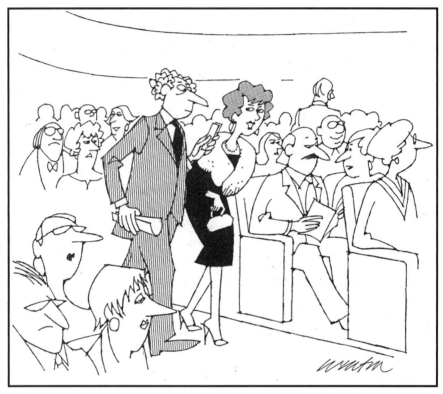

"I KNOW YOU'VE BEEN ON CALL TOO LONG WHEN THE TICKET SAYS SECTION C AND YOU READ IT AS C-SECTION."

hospitals, and all other types of healthcare services. A doctor practicing alone is less likely to be as efficient or, more important, as effective as doctors who practice in groups in an integrated system. More than that, since most consumers can't afford to pay for either a high monthly retainer fee or for all the healthcare they may need, they must have medical insurance to protect them from high out-of-pocket costs. Most doctors will do best who somehow continue to coordinate what they do with the usual ways doctors get paid by insurance companies.

Measuring quality is important and must start somewhere.

This is not to say that a solo physician is not able to provide the best medical care. It is simply very difficult. To provide the best medical care and thrive financially, this doctor would most likely have to link up with a large multi-specialty physician group that is committed to providing high-quality modern medicine and that bills insurance companies on behalf of its patients.

Technology—Help or Hindrance?

Most physicians today need better electronic systems to help them do their jobs. With fully integrated computer systems, doctors could keep up with breaking research, track each patient's medical history, and much more. But relatively few doctors have access to such state-of-the-art electronic systems. The cost of purchasing, implementing, and maintaining good electronic systems is far more than any one doctor alone can usually afford. This leaves most physicians dependent on the deeper pockets of insurance companies, large hospital systems, or large medical groups to supply and maintain electronic support systems.

Even when large organizations offer electronic systems and other support, doctors must often give up some of their independence to participate in or coordinate with these large organizations. A doctor may have to become salaried instead of being in business for himself or herself. Or he or she may have to cut the amount of time spent with each patient or in some other way make tough compromises.

Some doctors are leery of health systems that incorporate system-wide computerization. They feel that some of these systems focus on making profits, downplaying customer service or clinical quality. Many doctors find "selling their medical souls" to a health system too high a price for technological and other support. They often choose to continue working as they have in the past, rather than make any changes.

Frankly, even more distasteful to some of these physicians is the threat of being measured more closely against a standard of quality of care. It takes courage to move out of a safe position where the care you provide is not questioned into a system where quality is measured. This is especially true for doctors who mistrust the way systems measure or define quality. Nevertheless, measuring quality is important and must start somewhere.

Most physicians today need better electronic systems to help them do their jobs.

A Better System for Doctors

Much of this book has been dedicated to describing how the medical system needs to change to better serve the healthcare consumer. The following list describes the other side of the coin—changes that would benefit doctors and support them in providing the quality of care that consumers need and deserve.

- All physicians should be able to work in a setting that provides state-of-the-art electronic support systems. These systems should offer easy access to updated scientific evidence about the best available treatments for each type of medical problem. They should also provide easily accessible, detailed tracking of each patient's full medical history and records. Access to these systems should not require physicians to make unacceptable compromises in giving the best care to patients.

- Physicians should maintain the power to make independent decisions about each patient's care, *in partnership with the patient, and within the context of guidelines for high-quality care.*

- Physician income should reflect the high value of high-quality medical care. Physicians whose work leads to better health outcomes should be paid more.

Unfortunately, it is much easier to describe a better healthcare system from the physician's viewpoint than to figure out how to get there from here.

26 You *Can* Make a Difference in Your Healthcare

It is better to be making the news than taking it;
to be an actor rather than a critic.   —Winston Churchill

Whether you think you can or whether you think you can't
—you are right.   —Henry Ford

You miss 100% of the shots you never take.
                                        —Wayne Gretzki

In This Chapter...

- To get the best health possible, take charge of your healthcare and take ownership of your health.
- The specific steps you can take to combine wise lifestyle choices with being a wise healthcare consumer to maximize your health.

Now it's time to wrap things up so you can get to work. Whether you are in excellent health or in need of medical attention, your health is ultimately your responsibility. And, while many people take their health for granted—at least until they contract an illness or incur an injury—most of us cherish good health above most everything else. After all, without it, nearly every other part of life suffers.

The healthcare system that we've been discussing in these pages is intended to serve you—to support you as a consumer of healthcare services in maintaining good health—preventing you from getting ill, preserving your good health, and healing you when you're ailing. But you are the one who needs to be in charge—not the doctors or the insurance companies.

Three Key Points for Getting Better Care

So let's recap what you've read in the preceding pages. As bad as the system is, there's hope: Informed consumers are the primary catalysts for positive change. Every quality improvement made to the system will benefit consumers, so we all benefit by advocating positive change. To achieve all this, here are a few things to remember:

Whether you are in excellent health or in need of medical attention, your health is ultimately your responsibility.

1. Keep Learning

• Learn the language and structure of the healthcare industry, at least enough to be able to ask for what you need.

• Be willing to ask questions and search for information, and don't stop until you are satisfied with the answers.

2. Make Wise Choices

Choose plans that offer the following:

• Integrated networks of healthcare professionals who talk to one another about your situation and who coordinate all of your care.

• Customer-centered care that is focused on respect for you as a person and your well-being and convenience.

• Evidence of providers' high level of quality by participation in quality measurement surveys.

3. Take Charge

• Accept ownership of your health; don't abdicate to "experts," and don't expect medical care to protect you from disease if you are not willing to live a healthy lifestyle.

• Find out what your highest health risks are, based on your lifestyle and family history. Get help from your doctor and do your own research to figure out the diseases and health problems you are most likely to develop.

• Change your lifestyle as necessary to lower your health risks.

• Make sure to get all the appropriate health services and preventive care you should have, even if your doctor does not suggest it before you do.

• Be willing to challenge convention. Stop believing the myths.

• Speak up when you aren't being respected or when you need to make sure you are getting the best care.

Anecdotal vs. Scientific Evidence

There's one last, important thing I want to impart to you before we go: Please, for your own sake, don't be unduly swayed by anecdotal evidence!

For some reason, human beings seem to favor anecdotes over scientific evidence, such as statistical facts. Here's an example. Suppose I told you that, based on valid research, the chances of your surviving a certain type of surgery are only 20%. That sounds pretty bad. Most people would seriously look for alternatives to that surgery. Then suppose I told you about a wonderful woman I know who, with the same chances of survival, successfully had this surgery and fully recovered from her illness, and is today leading a full, normal, happy life. Your hope for being among the 20% survivors would likely increase by hearing this anecdote. That's just the way our brains seem to work. Does hearing the anecdote change your odds for surviving the surgery? No. Does the increased hope of survival increase your odds? Maybe, but should you base your entire decision on this increased hope? Probably not, unless the survival rate for alternatives to the surgery are even more grim.

This story serves as an illustration of how we may be basing many of our decisions about healthcare on anecdotes rather than on a logical evaluation of the facts. For example, let's say you need to choose a health plan and your neighbor tells you he had a bad experience with a health plan that is rated highly in multiple surveys. Is it logical for you to base your decision on your neighbor's experience rather than on the survey ratings? No.

It is true that "scientific" evidence, often presented in the form of statistics, can be swayed to show proof of whatever the presenter wants to prove. It is also true that the way something is measured can sway the statistical results and make facts appear true when they are not. The current "science" of measuring healthcare quality is in its infancy and does not always measure precisely what is intended. But measuring and comparing healthcare providers must start somewhere. We just need to keep this in mind when reviewing the statistics.

For your own sake, remember that human beings tend to be swayed by anecdotal evidence. Anecdotes can be useful in understanding issues. That's why I have included many anecdotal stories in this book. But as tools for making sound healthcare decisions, anecdotes cannot begin to compete with scientifically validated broad collections of evidence.

> As tools for making sound healthcare decisions, anecdotes cannot begin to compete with scientifically validated broad collections of evidence.

The Big Payoff for Being Thorough

Ultimately, the main benefit of making wise health decisions is your well-being—both physical and emotional. You can live with confidence that you and your family are receiving the best attention, whether you are in need right now or are simply taking preventive measures. With this peace of mind comes emotional calm, a serenity that accompanies confidence about your and your family's health.

This is where we part company. It has been a pleasure putting all this information together for you, and I wish you a rewarding adventure finding high-quality healthcare.

You have my sincerest wishes for the very best of good health and, in the event you do need medical attention of any kind, the most competent of support and the highest-quality treatment. May you live a long and disability-free life.

PART VII

APPENDICES:
RESOURCES TO ASSIST YOU IN
MAKING WISE CHOICES

Appendix A
General Sources of Information on Medical Issues

Appendix B
Sources of Quality Comparison Data

Please note that the resource data listed in the following
sections, as in the rest of the book, are accurate and the
best I can recommend as of the date this book is being
prepared for printing. Given the fast-changing nature of
healthcare, the resources or information could change at
any time.

Appendix A:
General Sources of Information on Medical Issues

Appendix A lists online and print resources where you can find information about specific diseases or conditions as well as about staying healthy.

Online Resources

The U.S. Department of Health and Human Services offers some advice for evaluating a healthcare website.[1] Before trusting the information on a site, ask yourself:

• Does the website clearly state its purpose and its sponsors, and does it separate advertising and sales from health information?

• Does it get its information from reliable sources and keep that information up-to-date?

• Does the site tell me what information it collects about me and how that information will be used and protected?

If you can't answer "yes" to these questions, look somewhere else for medical advice.

Medical Library Association Top Ten Recommended Websites

The Medical Library Association (MLA) was founded a century ago "to encourage the improvement and increase of public medical libraries." This highly respected organization provides a carefully screened, continuously monitored and updated list of "Top Ten" Most Useful Consumer Health Websites on its own website at *www.mlanet.org*. Also on the MLA website are additional lists of websites on cancer, diabetes, and heart disease. MLA evaluates websites based on the following criteria: credibility, sponsorship/authorship, content, audience, currency, disclosure, purpose, links, design, interactivity, and disclaimers. At the time this book was printed, the following websites were on MLA's "Top Ten" list. Check the MLA website for updates to this list. Note that this list is in alphabetical order by organization name, not by comparative value of the site.

Centers for Disease Control and Prevention
(www.cdc.gov)
This agency of the Department of Health and Human Services is dedicated to promoting "health and quality of life by pre-

venting and controlling disease, injury, and disability." Of special interest are the resources about diseases, conditions, and other special topics arranged under "Health Topics A to Z" and "Travelers' Health." Information is also available in Spanish.

Healthfinder

(www.healthfinder.gov)

This site is the healthcare portal of the U.S. Department of Health and Human Services. The goal of the website is "to improve consumer access to selected health information from government agencies, their many partner organizations, and other reliable sources that serve the public interest." It is a gateway to hundreds of reliable online health publications, databases, websites, support groups, self-help groups, government agencies, and non-profit organizations. The developer and sponsor of this site is the Office of Disease Prevention and Health Promotion, Department of Health and Human Services, with other agencies that also can be accessed via the site. Access to resources on the site is also available in Spanish.

Health Web

(http://healthweb.org)

This is a site established by librarians and information professionals from major academic medical institutions in the Midwest. You can search the site either by entering search terms or by selecting one of the many alphabetically listed medical subjects. When a medical subject is selected, you can go into more depth by using the left side of the screen to select narrower subjects or categories. The site also provides "User Guides" developed to help consumers use Internet resources more effectively.

HIV InSite

(http://hivinsite.ucsf.edu)

This is a project of the University of California San Francisco (UCSF) AIDS Research Institute. Designed as a gateway to in-depth information about particular aspects of HIV/AIDS, it provides numerous links to many authoritative sources. Subjects are arranged in "Key Topics" and the site may also be searched by keywords. Many items are provided in full text, and information is available in English and Spanish.

Mayo Clinic

(www.mayoclinic.com)

This site is an extension of the Mayo Clinic's commitment to provide health education to patients and the general public.

Editors of the site include more than 2,000 physicians, scientists, writers, and educators at the Mayo Clinic, a non-profit institution with more than 100 years of history in patient care, medical research, and education. A new format, which recently debuted, has added interactive tools to assist consumers in managing their health.

Medem
(http://medem.com)
This site, launched in the fall of 2000, is a project of the leading medical societies in the United States. Some of the founding societies include the American Medical Association, the American Academy of Pediatrics, and the American College of Obstetricians and Gynecologists. The site was developed to provide "a trusted online source for credible, comprehensive, and clinical healthcare information, and secure, confidential communications." The "Medical Library" is divided into four major categories: Life Stages, Diseases and Conditions, Therapies and Health Strategies, and Health and Society.

MEDLINEplus
(http://medlineplus.gov)
This is a consumer-oriented website established by the National Library of Medicine, the world's largest biomedical library and creator of the MEDLINE database. An alphabetical list of "Health Topics" consists of more than 300 specific diseases, conditions, and wellness issues. Each Health Topic page contains links to authoritative information on that subject, as well as an optional link to a pre-formulated MEDLINE search that provides journal article citations on the subject. Additional resources include physician and hospital directories, several online medical dictionaries, and consumer drug information available by generic or brand name.

National Women's Health Information Center
(www.4women.gov)
This site is a gateway to selected women's health information resources. Its purpose is to provide a single site on the Web where women can locate reliable, timely resources about "prevention, diagnosis, and treatment of the illnesses and health conditions that affect them." It is sponsored by the U.S. Public Health Service's Office on Women's Health and provides access to a variety of women's federal and private-sector resources. An alphabetical "Health Topics" menu makes searching easy. Information is available in both English and Spanish.

NOAH: New York Online Access to Health

(www.noah-health.org)

This is a unique collection of local, state, and federal health resources for consumers. NOAH's mission is "to provide high-quality, full-text information for consumers that is accurate, timely, relevant, and unbiased." Information is arranged in alphabetical "Health Topics," which are then narrowed to include definitions, care and treatment, and lists of information resources. Information is available in both English and Spanish, and the majority of items are provided in full text.

Oncolink®: A University of Pennsylvania Cancer Center Resource

(http://oncolink.upenn.edu)

This site provides information on the various forms of cancer and issues of interest to cancer patients and their families. The site may be searched by keywords or by menus, including disease-oriented menus and medical specialty-oriented menus. Major areas covered are cancer causes, symptom management, clinical trials, psychosocial support, cancer FAQs (frequently asked questions), and global resources for cancer information.

Print Resources

The following list includes print periodicals as well as the two books heavily referenced in *Surviving Healthcare* that were published by the Institute of Medicine to report to the nation on healthcare quality issues. You can find out more about each of the periodicals at your local library. If you have access to the Internet, you may also find information about many of them by doing a search using your favorite search engine, for example, Google, Yahoo!, or Dogpile. You can get copies of the Institute of Medicine books at your local bookstore (ask the bookstore to place a special order if they don't have copies on hand) or through online booksellers.

American Fitness

Consumer Reports On Health

Harvard Health Letter

Harvard Men's Health Watch

Harvard Mental Health Letter

Harvard Women's Health Watch

The Johns Hopkins Medical Letter Health After 50

Mayo Clinic Women's Healthsource

Tufts University Health And Nutrition Letter

University of California, Berkeley, Wellness Letter

Committee on Quality Health Care in America, Institute of Medicine. *Crossing the Quality Chasm: A New Health System for the 21st Century.* Washington, D.C.: National Academy Press, 2001.

L.T. Kohn, J.M. Corrigan, M.S. Donaldson, eds. *To Err Is Human: Building a Safer Health System.* Washington, D.C.: National Academy Press, 2000.

Appendix B:
Sources of Quality Comparison Data

Appendix B lists websites where you can find data comparing health plans, hospitals, and medical groups. I have also provided a source of information on doctors: the National Committee for Quality Assurance (NCQA) lists, which report doctors participating in the Diabetes and (soon) Heart/Stroke recognition programs. Only a few resources provide good quality comparison information on medical groups, and this information is limited to certain parts of the country.

Because little information is available for fee-for-service and related types of plans, most of the sites listed here provide information on rating HMOs only. Only the NCQA and Health Pages listings below give information on PPO ratings.

It is unfortunate that there is limited useful data currently available for rating medical providers, but as the emphasis on quality improvement expands, more resources will focus on collecting and publishing valid comparison information. I hope and assume the list below will be out-of-date soon. Watch for new credible sources of provider evaluation. In the meantime, in the absence of good comparison data in most parts of the country, it is important to learn about the elements of quality and to look for them.

American Accreditation Healthcare Commission, Inc. (URAC)
(www.urac.org)
URAC (which used to stand for Utilization Review Accreditation Commission but which is now just an acronym), also known as the American Accreditation Healthcare Commission, is a non-profit organization that establishes standards for the healthcare industry. Founded in 1990, URAC provides independent, neutral evaluation of many types of healthcare organizations, including hospitals, HMOs, PPOs, and third-party administrators and provider groups. Accreditation adds value to these programs by providing a seal of approval from an outside source and by promoting quality improvement within the organization as part of the accreditation process.

In 2001, URAC also began accrediting health-related websites through its Health Web Site Accreditation Review program. Web accreditation requires that providers of health content, tools, and website services meet 53 specific standards.

HealthScope (California)

(www.healthscope.org)

The Pacific Business Group on Health sponsors this site, where California consumers can find good information to help them select high-quality health plans, hospitals, and medical groups. The site also provides health resources.

The Health Plan portion of this site rates HMOs by county. The ratings provide a large volume of easy-to-understand information, particularly in the Summary category. Each category includes an At a Glance compilation of the results for all of that category's factors.

The Hospitals portion of this site provides two reports for the hospitals in each California county: General Care or Heart Care.

Joint Commission on Accreditation of Healthcare Organizations (JCAHO)

(www.jcaho.org)

The Joint Commission on Accreditation of Healthcare Organizations evaluates and accredits more than 17,000 healthcare organizations and programs in the United States. An independent, non-profit organization, JCAHO is the nation's predominant standards-setting body for hospitals. Since 1951, JCAHO has developed state-of-the-art, professionally-based standards and has evaluated the compliance of hospitals against these benchmarks. In recent times, JCAHO has expanded its reviews to other types of healthcare provider organizations, and now includes hospitals, healthcare networks, home care organizations, nursing homes, assisted living facilities, behavioral healthcare organizations, ambulatory care providers, and clinical laboratories. JCAHO accreditation is recognized nationwide as a symbol of quality that reflects an organization's commitment to meeting certain performance standards.

Currently, about 50% of JCAHO's hospital standards are directly related to safety. These standards address issues such as the implementation of patient safety programs, the responsibility of organization leadership to create a culture of safety, the prevention of medical errors through the prospective analysis and redesign of vulnerable patient systems (e.g., the ordering, preparation, and dispensing of medications), and the hospital's responsibility to tell a patient if he or she has been harmed by the care provided. The General Public area of the JCAHO website contains a patient safety section with helpful information for consumers.

National Committee for Quality Assurance's (NCQA) HealthChoices

(www.healthchoices.org)

HealthChoices is the NCQA's consumer-focused website. Here you will find information to help you select from among hundreds of managed care plans (HMO/POS and PPO) that care for commercially insured individuals and Medicare and Medicaid beneficiaries. Based on a rigorous evaluation of clinical quality, member satisfaction, and a comprehensive assessment of key systems and processes, the Report Card can help you answer questions about health plans that would be difficult or impossible to answer on your own: Does this health plan provide good customer service? Will I have access to care I need? Does the plan check doctors' qualifications? If I get sick, which plan will take better care of me?

Access this website to create a customized report card that shows results for the health plan or plans in your state or ZIP code.

National Committee for Quality Assurance's (NCQA) Quality Compass (national)

(www.ncqa.org/Info/QualityCompass)

Quality Compass is the NCQA's comprehensive national database of health plans survey results. It contains plan-specific, comparative, and descriptive information on the performance of hundreds of managed care organizations—providing benefits managers, health plans, consultants, the media, and others with the ability to conduct a detailed market analysis. Whether you are interested in data for competitive analysis or marketing, or to help select a health plan, Quality Compass is an invaluable resource.

State of California's Office of the Patient Advocate (OPA)

(www.opa.ca.gov)

The State of California, in conjunction with Sapient Corporation and the Pacific Business Group on Health, analyzes publicly reported quality information about California HMOs and provides the results to consumers in an easy-to-use format on the website of the state's Office of the Patient Advocate. HMOs are rated and compared on how well they handle diabetes, heart care, mental health, women's health, and several other aspects of their care and services. Also on this website is a comparison of the largest medical groups in the state, county by county, also in an easily usable format.

The Leapfrog Group (urban/regional)

(www.leapfroggroup.org)

This site includes results of the ongoing Leapfrog Group Hospital Patient Safety Survey. The survey evaluates urban acute-care hospitals on their efforts to reduce preventable medical mistakes. The survey currently measures the care of seven high-risk conditions. Research indicates that meeting the standards for patient safety for these conditions saves many lives and prevents many serious medication errors each year. The conditions are listed and the standards are outlined on the website.

At the time of this book's printing, Leapfrog's outreach focuses on the following regions: Atlanta, Georgia; California; Central Florida; Colorado; Dallas–Fort Worth, Texas; Hampton Roads, Virginia; Illinois; Kansas City, Missouri; Maine; Massachusetts; Memphis, Tennessee; Metro New York, New York; Michigan; Minnesota; East Tennessee; New Jersey; Rochester, New York; Savannah, Georgia; Seattle, Washington; St. Louis, Missouri; Wisconsin; and Wichita, Kansas. The majority of the information on the site comes from these regions. Some hospitals outside of these areas are now submitting their data to Leapfrog, reflecting a growing awareness of the need for sharing quality data with the public.

Endnotes

Introduction

[1] L.T. Kohn, J.M. Corrigan, and M.S. Donaldson, eds., *To Err is Human: Building a Safer Health System* (Washington, D.C.: National Academy Press, 2000).

[2] Committee on Quality Health Care in America, Institute of Medicine, *Crossing the Quality Chasm: A New Health System for the 21ˢᵗ Century* (Washington, D.C.: National Academy Press, 2001);

Chapter 1

[1] L.T. Kohn, J.M. Corrigan, and M.S. Donaldson, eds., *To Err is Human: Building a Safer Health System* (Washington, D.C.: National Academy Press, 2000).

[2] National Committee for Quality Assurance, "The State of Health Care Quality: 2003." (2003) Report available at *www.ncqa.org*.

[3] E.A. McGlynn et al., "The Quality of Health Care Delivered to Adults in the United States," *New England Journal of Medicine* Vol. 348, No. 26 (June 26, 2003), 2635-2645.

[4] M.A. Schuster, E.A. McGlynn and R.H. Brook, "How Good is the Quality of Health Care in the United States?" *Milbank Memorial Quarterly*, Vol. 76, No. 4, 1998, 517-563.

[5] R.A. Hahn et al., "Excess Deaths from Nine Chronic Diseases in the United States, 1986," *Journal of the American Medical Association* Vol. 264, No. 20 (November 28, 1990), 2654-2660.

[6] Midwest Business Group on Health in collaboration with the Juram Institute, Inc., and The Severyn Group, Inc., "Reducing the Costs of Poor-Quality Health Care" (2003).

[7] A.M. Minino and B.L. Smith, "Deaths: Preliminary Data for 2000," *National Vital Statistics Reports* Vol. 49, No. 12 (Hyattsville, Maryland: National Center for Health Statistics, 2001).

[8] C. Zhan and M.R. Miller, "Excess Length of Stay, Charges, and Mortality Attributable to Medical Injuries During Hospitalization," *Journal of the American Medical Association*, Vol. 290, No. 14 (October 8, 2003), 1868-1874.

[9] Agency for Healthcare Research and Quality, "Reducing and Preventing Adverse Drug Events to Decrease Hospital Costs," *Research in Action* Issue 1, publication number 01-0020 (March 2001).

[10] In three-tier drug copayment plans, you pay the lowest copay amount for generic drugs, the next highest amount for brand-name drugs on your plan's "formulary" list, and the highest copay amount for brand-name drugs that are not on your plan's formulary list. For example, you might pay $10 for a 30-day supply of a prescribed generic drug, $20 for a

30-day supply of a prescribed brand-name drug that is on the formulary list, and $30 for a 30-day supply of a prescribed brand-name drug that is not on your plan's formulary list. The trick for the consumer, to pay as little as possible for prescribed drugs, is to always get your physician to prescribe a generic drug if one is available that meets your needs. If a generic is not available, let your doctor know which of the brand-name drugs that will meet your needs is on your plan's formulary list. Most plans make their current formulary list available on their website. If you don't have Internet access, or if the list is not available or is difficult to find online, try calling the member services phone number for your plan for assistance.

Chapter 3

[1] Institute for the Future, *Health and Health Care 2010: The Forecast, The Challenge* (Princeton, New Jersey: Jossey-Bass, 2003), 23.

Chapter 4

[1] W.C. Winkelmayer, MD, ScD, et al., "Preventive Health Care Measures Before and After Start of Renal Replacement Therapy," *Journal of General Internal Medicine* 17 (August 2002), 588-595.

[2] E.A. McGlynn et al., "The Quality of Health Care Delivered to Adults in the United States," *New England Journal of Medicine* Vol. 348, No. 26 (June 26, 2003), 2635-2645.

[3] A.P. Legoretta et al., "Variations in Managing Asthma: Experience at the Medical Group Level in California," *American Journal of Managed Care* 6 (2000), 445–453; C.M. Clark et al., "Promoting Early Diagnosis and Treatment of Type 2 Diabetes," *Journal of the American Medical Association* Vol. 284, No. 3 (July 19, 2000), 363-365.

Chapter 5

[1] From television broadcast: "CNN Your Health," aired July 27, 2002, 14:30 ET. Transcript available at *www.cnn.com/TRANSCRIPTS/0207/27/yh.00.html*.

[2] Much information in this section comes from an excellent report issued by the Midwest Business Group on Health (MBGH) titled "How We Choose Doctors—What Is and What Could Be," published in 2000. You can get a copy of this report by visiting *www.mbgh.org* and looking under Publications.

Chapter 6

[1] Committee on Quality Health Care in America, Institute of Medicine, *Crossing the Quality Chasm: A New Health System for the 21st Century* (Washington, D.C.: National Academy Press, 2001);

[2] Ibid.

[3] These suggestions have been compiled from the following websites, which are good sources for additional suggestions/information about how to talk with and work with your doctor:
www.ahcpr.gov/consumer/quicktips/doctalk.htm

www.plainsense.com/Health/General/doctalk.htm
www.elfstrom.com/arthritis/appointments.html
www.aarp.org/confacts/health/talkdr.html
www.ama-assn.org/insight/spec_con/patient/pat081.pdf

Chapter 7

[1] R.A. Hahn et al., "Excess Deaths from Nine Chronic Diseases in the United States, 1986," *Journal of the American Medical Association* Vol. 264, No. 20 (November 28, 1990), 2654-2660.

[2] A.V. Chobanian, MD, et al., "The Seventh Report of the Joint National Committee on Prevention, Detection, Evaluation, and Treatment of High Blood Pressure," *Journal of the American Medical Association* Vol. 289, No. 19 (May 21, 2003), 2560.

[3] Ibid.

[4] Ibid.

[5] Ibid.

[6] Ibid.

[7] L.S. Phillips et al., "Clinical Inertia," *Annals of Internal Medicine* 135 (2001), 825-834.

[8] Chobanian, Op. cit.

[9] Agency for Healthcare Research and Quality, "About USPSTF: The New U.S. Preventive Services Task Force" (February 2002). Report available at *www.ahrq.gov/clinic/uspstfab.htm*.

[10] Committee on Quality Health Care in America, Institute of Medicine, Op. cit., adapted from Table A-1, 250-257.

[11] A.B. Coffield et al., "Priorities Among Recommended Clinical Preventive Services," *American Journal of Preventive Medicine* Vol. 21, No. 1 (July, 2001), 1-9.

[12] B.F. Crabtree, W.L. Miller, and K.C. Stange, "Understanding Practice From the Ground Up," *Journal of Family Practice* Vol. 50, No. 10 (October 2001), 881-887.

[13] Phillips, Op. cit.

[14] Coffield, Op. cit.

Chapter 8

[1] R.N. Remen, MD, "Health, Happiness, and the Well-Lived Life: A Doctor's Prescription," *Oprah The Magazine* (January 2003), 138.

[2] Institute for the Future, *Health and Health Care 2010: The Forecast, The Challenge* (Princeton, New Jersey: Jossey-Bass, 2003), 23.

[3] *Business Wire* (Salt Lake City: August 26, 2002).

[4] AgePage (2003) *www.nia.nih.gov/health/agepages/exercise.htm*, 1.

[5] National Center for Chronic Disease Prevention and Health Promotion, "Preventing Obesity and Chronic Diseases Through Good Nutrition and Physical Activity," U.S. Centers for Disease Control and Prevention (2003) (*www.cdc.gov/nccdphp/pe_factsheets/pe_pa.htm*), 1.

[6] Ibid, 3.

[7] Ibid, 1.

[8] Healthier U.S. (2003) *www.healthierus.gov*, home page.

[9] National Center for Chronic Disease Prevention and Health Promotion, Op. cit.

[10] Ibid.

[11] K.B. Eden et al., "Does Counseling by Clinicians Improve Physical Activity?: A Summary of the Evidence for the U.S. Preventive Services Task Force," *Annals of Internal Medicine* 137 (2002), 208-215.

[12] U.S. Dept. of Health and Human Services, 1996.

[13] Eden, Op. cit.

[14] Centers for Disease Control and Prevention, "Can Inactivity Hurt My Health?" *www.cdc.gov/nccdphp/dnpa/physical/importance/inactivity.htm* (Pratt, Macera, & Blanton, 1999).

[15] From television broadcast: CNN, aired June 22, 2002, 14:30 ET. Transcript available at *www.cnn.com/TRANSCRIPTS/0206/22/yh.00.html*.

[16] National Center for Chronic Disease Prevention and Health Promotion, Op. cit.

[17] C. Farrell, "The Economics of a Fatter America," *Business Week Online* (February 28, 2003).

[18] V.W. Chang, MD, MA, and N.A. Christakis, MD, PhD, MPH, "Extent and Determinants of Discrepancy Between Self-Evaluations of Weight Status and Clinical Standards," *Journal of General Internal Medicine* 16(8) (August, 2001), 538-543.

[19] Healthier U.S., Op. cit.

[20] N. Hellmich, "Obesity in America Is Worse Than Ever: 6 in 10 Are Overweight; Health Fallout Is Feared," *USA Today* (October 10, 2002), 1A.

[21] G.L. Blackburn, Chairman of Nutrition Medicine at Harvard Medical School, as quoted in S. Squires, "Study Finds That in U.S., 1 in 3 Are Obese," *Washington Post* (October 9, 2002).

[22] These guidelines derive substantially from the Mayo Clinic's "Guide for Healthy Eating," a medical essay supplement to the *Mayo Clinic Health Letter* (Mayo Foundation for Medical Education and Research, 2002).

[23] Healthier U.S., Op. cit.

[24] The federal Agency for Healthcare Research and Quality, reported in *USA Today* (December 24, 2002), and at the Agency's website *www.ahrq.gov/clinic/cps3dix.htm*.

[25] Remen, Op. cit., pp. 136-139.

Chapter 10

[1] D. Vaughan, *The Challenger Launch Decision: Risky Technology, Culture, and Deviance at NASA* (Chicago and London: The University of Chicago Press, 1996).

[2] California Medicine Roundtable, "Understanding Healthcare Quality," *California Medicine Roundtable Special Supplement* (June/July 1999), Q11; E.A. McGlynn et al., "The Quality of Health Care Delivered to Adults in the United States," *New England Journal of Medicine* Vol. 348, No. 26 (June 26, 2003), 2635-2645.; L. Casalino et al., "External Incentives, Information Technology, and Organized Processes to Improve Health Care Quality for Patients with Chronic Diseases," *Journal of the American Medical Association* Vol. 289, No. 4 (January 22-29, 2003), 434-441.

[3] Based on estimates by medical experts. No confirmation of this percentage is available.

[4] Office of Technology Assessment of the Congress of the United States, "The Impact of Randomized Clinical Trials on Health Policy and Medical Practice," *Background Paper OTA-BP-H-22* (Washington, D.C.: U.S. Government Printing Office, August 1983).

[5] M. Cabana, MD, MPH, et al., "Why Don't Physicians Follow Clinical Practice Guidelines? A Framework for Improvement," *Journal of the American Medical Association*, 282(15), October 20, 1999), 1458-1465.

Chapter 11

[1] L.T. Kohn, J.M. Corrigan, and M.S. Donaldson, eds., *To Err is Human: Building a Safer Health System* (Washington, D.C.: National Academy Press, 2000).

[2] C. Zhan and M.R. Miller, "Excess Length of Stay, Charges, and Mortality Attributable to Medical Injuries During Hospitalization," *Journal of the American Medical Association*, Vol. 290, No. 14 (October 8, 2003), 1868-1874.

[3] Agency for Healthcare Research and Quality, "Reducing and Preventing Adverse Drug Events to Decrease Hospital Costs," *Research in Action* Issue 1, publication number 01-0020 (March 2001).

[4] Consumers Union of U.S., Inc., "HMO or PPO: Picking a Managed-Care Plan," *Consumer Reports* (October 2003).

Chapter 12

[1] Committee on Quality Health Care in America, Institute of Medicine, *Crossing the Quality Chasm: A New Health System for the 21st Century* (Washington, D.C.: National Academy Press, 2001).

[2] F. Chen, MD, M.P.H., L.A. Rhodes, Ph.D., and L.A. Green, MD, "Family Physicians' Personal Experiences of Their Fathers' Healthcare," *Journal of Family Practice* Vol. 50, No. 9 (September 2001), 762-766.

[3] Casalino, Op. cit.; T.G. Rundall et al., "As Good As It Gets?: Chronic Care Management in Nine Leading US Physician Organisations," *British Medical Journal* Vol. 325, Issue 7370 (October 26, 2002), 958.

Chapter 14

[1] D.M. Studdert, LLB, ScD, MPH, and C.R. Gresenz, PhD, "Enrollee Appeals of Preservice Coverage Denials at 2 Health Maintenance Organizations," *Journal of the American Medical Association* Vol. 289, No. 7 (February 19, 2003), 864-870.

Chapter 15

[1] S.M. Shortell et al., "Integrating Health Care Delivery," *Health Forum Journal* Vol. 43, Issue 6 (Nov/Dec 2000), 35-39.

[2] S.M. Shortell et al, *Remaking Health Care in America, 2nd Edition* (San Francisco: Jossey-Bass, 2000), 1-17.

Chapter 16

[1] H. Taylor and R. Leitman, eds., "eHealth's Influence Continues to Grow as Usage of the Internet by Physicians and Patients Increases," *Health Care News* Vol. 3, No. 6 (April 17, 2003).

[2] S. Fox and D. Fallows, "Internet Health Resources: Health Searches and Email Have Become More Commonplace, But There is Room for Improvement in Searches and Overall Internet Access," *Pew Internet & American Life Project* (Washington, D.C.: July 2003).

[3] Kevin Fickenscher, MD, quoted in Jill Elswick, "Resources Growing For Employee-Consumers," *Employee Benefit News* (May 2002).

[4] RAND Health, "Proceed with Caution: A Report on the Quality of Health Information on the Internet" (California HealthCare Foundation, May 2001).

[5] M. Edlin, "Electronic Medicine: Pilot Programs Define Uses and Payment for Online Consultations," *Managed Healthcare Executive* (March 1, 2003).

[6] S.M. Shortell et al., "Integrating Health Care Delivery," *Health Forum Journal* Vol. 43, Issue 6 (Nov/Dec 2000), 35-39.

[7] Institute of Medicine, *Leadership By Example: Coordinating Government Roles in Improving Health Care Policy* (Washington, D.C.: National Academy Press, 2002).

[8] H. Taylor and R. Leitman, eds., "Why Not Spend More on Health Care?" *Harris Interactive Health Care News* Vol. 3, No. 12 (July 7, 2003).

[9] P. Aspden et al., eds., Committee on Data Standards for Patient Safety, Institute of Medicine, *Patient Safety: Achieving a New Standard for Care* (Washington D.C.: National Academy Press, 2003).

Chapter 18

[1] M.L. Millenson, *Demanding Medical Excellence* (Chicago and London: The University of Chicago Press, 1999).

[2] California Health Decisions, Inc., *Public Values and Perspectives on Managed Care* (October 1998).

[3] H.H. Schauffler et al., "Differences in the Kinds of Problems Consumers Report in Staff/Group Health Maintenance Organizations, Independent Practice Association/Network Health Maintenance Organizations, and Preferred Provider Organizations in California," *Medical Care* Vol. 39, Issue 1 (January 2001), 15-25.

[4] Consumers Union of U.S., Inc., "HMO or PPO: Picking a Managed-Care Plan," *Consumer Reports* (October 2003).

Chapter 19

[1] Consumers Union of U.S., Inc., "HMO or PPO: Picking a Managed-Care Plan," *Consumer Reports* (October 2003).

Chapter 22

[1] The Kaiser Family Foundation and Health Research and Educational Trust, "2003 Employer Health Benefits Survey" (The Henry J. Kaiser Family Foundation, September 2003).

[2] *Reuters*, February 7, 2003, as reported in the *Chicago Tribune*, same date. According to the U.S. Bureau of Labor Statistics, wage costs for the fourth quarter of 2002 increased by 0.4%, while the costs of employee benefits, primarily driven by increases in healthcare benefit costs, rose by an average of 1.3% over the same period.

[3] J. Elswick, "Employers Push to Change Health Behaviors," *Employee Benefit News* (August 2003).

[4] Midwest Business Group on Health in collaboration with the Juram Institute, Inc., and The Severyn Group, Inc., "Reducing the Costs of Poor-Quality Health Care" (2003).

[5] Forrester Research, Inc., as reported by Atlantic Information Services (February 5, 2003).

[6] Plunkett Research Ltd., "Plunkett's Health Care Industry Trends and Statistics," Summary (2003), 11.

Chapter 23

[1] The Kaiser Family Foundation and Health Research and Educational Trust, "2003 Employer Health Benefits Survey" (The Henry J. Kaiser Family Foundation, September 2003).

[2] U.S. Bureau of Labor Statistics (2002).

[3] The Kaiser Family Foundation, Op cit.

[4] Ibid.

[5] Plunkett Research Ltd., "Plunkett's Health Care Industry Trends and Statistics," Summary (2003), 8.

[6] D.R. Powell, "How to Achieve an ROI on Your Health Care Dollars," *Employee Benefits Journal, International Foundation of Employee Benefit Plans* Vol. 27, No. 1 (March 2002), 24-27.

[7] Midwest Business Group on Health in collaboration with the Juram Institute, Inc., and The Severyn Group, Inc., "Reducing the Costs of Poor-Quality Health Care" (2003).

[8] G.F. Anderson et al., "It's the Prices, Stupid: Why the United States Is So Different From Other Countries," *Health Affairs* Vol. 22, No. 3 (May 2003), 89-105.

[9] E.A. Finkelstein, I.C. Fiebelkorn, and G. Wang, "National Medical Spending Attributable to Overweight and Obesity: How Much, and Who's Paying?" *Health Affairs* (Bethesda, MD: Web Exclusive, Project Hope, May 2003).

Chapter 24

[1] G. Cowley et al., "Health For Life: Now, 'Integrative' Care," *Newsweek* (December 2, 2002).

[2] According to the National Institutes of Health, as reported in "Here's to Your Health!" *Oprah The Magazine* (January 2003), 145.

Chapter 25

[1] This is the story of a friend's doctor.

Appendix A

[1] John Batteiger, "Look Carefully at Health Care Sites," *San Francisco Chronicle* (June 24, 2001), E-3, E-5.

Index

Important Caution to the Reader

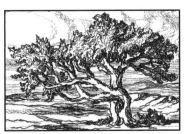

CHESTNUT RIDGE BOOKS

Quick Order Form

Fax orders: (775) 369-5450

Telephone orders: (800) 285-7307

Email orders: orders@SurvivingHealthcare.com

Postal orders: Chestnut Ridge Books
2269 Chestnut Street, #119
San Francisco, CA 94123-2600, USA

Please send ___ copies of *Surviving Healthcare* at $19.95 each

Name: _____

Address:_____

City:_____State:_____Zip: _____

Telephone: _____

Email address: _____

Sales tax: please add $1.50 per book for books shipped to California addresses

Shipping

U.S. $5.00 for first book, $2.00 for each additional book

Outside USA please e-mail for shipping rates *orders@SurvivingHealthcare.com*

Payment: ❏ Check   ❏ Credit Card:
❏ Visa   ❏ MasterCard   ❏ AMEX   ❏ Discover

Card number: _____

Name on card: _____

Exp. Date:_____ Signature _____

ORDER TOTAL: $_____